T0312734

Drug Compounding for Veterinary Professionals

Lauren R. Eichstadt Forsythe, PharmD, DICVP
Pharmacy Service Head
Clinical Assistant Professor – Department of Veterinary Clinical Medicine
University of Illinois at Urbana-Champaign
College of Veterinary Medicine
Veterinary Teaching Hospital
1008 West Hazelwood | M/C 004
Urbana, IL

Alexandria E. Gochenauer, PharmD, DICVP
Clinical Staff Pharmacist
University of Illinois at Urbana-Champaign
College of Veterinary Medicine
Veterinary Teaching Hospital
1008 West Hazelwood | M/C 004
Urbana, IL

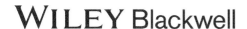

WILEY Blackwell

Copyright © 2023 by John Wiley & Sons, Inc. All rights reserved.

Published by John Wiley & Sons, Inc., Hoboken, New Jersey.
Published simultaneously in Canada.

No part of this publication may be reproduced, stored in a retrieval system, or transmitted in any form or by any means, electronic, mechanical, photocopying, recording, scanning, or otherwise, except as permitted under Section 107 or 108 of the 1976 United States Copyright Act, without either the prior written permission of the Publisher, or authorization through payment of the appropriate per-copy fee to the Copyright Clearance Center, Inc., 222 Rosewood Drive, Danvers, MA 01923, (978) 750-8400, fax (978) 750-4470, or on the web at www.copyright.com. Requests to the Publisher for permission should be addressed to the Permissions Department, John Wiley & Sons, Inc., 111 River Street, Hoboken, NJ 07030, (201) 748-6011, fax (201) 748-6008, or online at http://www.wiley.com/go/permission.

Trademarks: Wiley and the Wiley logo are trademarks or registered trademarks of John Wiley & Sons, Inc. and/or its affiliates in the United States and other countries and may not be used without written permission. All other trademarks are the property of their respective owners. John Wiley & Sons, Inc. is not associated with any product or vendor mentioned in this book.

Limit of Liability/Disclaimer of Warranty: While the publisher and author have used their best efforts in preparing this book, they make no representations or warranties with respect to the accuracy or completeness of the contents of this book and specifically disclaim any implied warranties of merchantability or fitness for a particular purpose. No warranty may be created or extended by sales representatives or written sales materials. The advice and strategies contained herein may not be suitable for your situation. You should consult with a professional where appropriate. Further, readers should be aware that websites listed in this work may have changed or disappeared between when this work was written and when it is read. Neither the publisher nor authors shall be liable for any loss of profit or any other commercial damages, including but not limited to special, incidental, consequential, or other damages.

For general information on our other products and services or for technical support, please contact our Customer Care Department within the United States at (800) 762-2974, outside the United States at (317) 572-3993 or fax (317) 572-4002.

Wiley also publishes its books in a variety of electronic formats. Some content that appears in print may not be available in electronic formats. For more information about Wiley products, visit our web site at www.wiley.com.

Library of Congress Cataloging-in-Publication Data applied for

Paperback ISBN: 9781119764960

Cover Design: Wiley
Cover Image: Courtesy of Alexandria Gochenauer

Set in 9.5/12.5pt STIXTwoText by Straive, Pondicherry, India

SKY10049058_061323

**Drug Compounding
for Veterinary Professionals**

Dedication

Lauren R. Eichstadt Forsythe: For my husband who always encourages me to push beyond my limits, and for my mom for serving as my inspiration for the questions plaguing veterinarians outside of academia.

Alexandria E. Gochenauer: To each and every person who has supported me along the way during my journey to becoming a veterinary pharmacist.

Contents

Foreword

It is a pleasure to offer this introduction to Nonsterile and Sterile Compounding for the Veterinary Practitioner.

Compounding of drugs administered for the prevention or treatment of diseases in animals has always been a critically important aspect of veterinary medicine. The number of drugs approved by the Food and Drug Administration (FDA) for the treatment of animals is limited. Approval is challenging given the diversity of species (thus physiology and pathology), patient numbers (e.g. herds and lab animals) and facilities (e.g. farms, wildlife, zoo, or marine facilities). Compounding offers the opportunity for the administration of formulations customized for the individual patient, regardless of the situation, in the absence of approved drugs. The use of compounded drugs by veterinarians is protected by law through the Animal Medicinal Drug Use Clarification Act of 1994 (AMDUCA). The Act not only delineates conditions under which veterinarians can use compounded drugs, but it also legalizes the act of compounding by veterinarians. It is the responsibility of the FDA's Center for Veterinary Medicine to regulate the law and, specifically, the compounded drugs that are considered unapproved new drugs. However, the path to regulation by the Center for Veterinary Medicine, delineated in nonlegally binding guidance documents for industry, has been difficult. This partially reflects the lack of clarity in the law, leading to differences in interpretation between compounders and regulatory agencies.

Despite this lack of clarity – or perhaps because of it – the last two decades have been accompanied by a marked increase in the use of compounded products by veterinarians. This increase likely reflects improved diagnostics and a greater expectation of owners regarding the delivery of state-of-the-art medical care to their animals. The promotion of commercial compounded products by pharmacies or outsourcing facilities has facilitated the access of these products. On the one hand, this expansion of compounding has had a positive influence on the delivery of state-of-the-art care for veterinary patients. But challenges also have emerged, ranging from the compounding of products that mimic approved drugs to the promotion of novel and sophisticated delivery systems that are not supported by scientific evidence of safety or efficacy.

The FDA perceives that compounded drugs present a greater risk of adversity than approved formulations, and this is particularly true if the end result of compounding is a poor product. Adversities can include too much drug, too little drug, poor delivery, or the presence of unanticipated chemicals. Although the use of compounded preparations by veterinarians has increased, the skill sets and knowledge base needed to effectively prescribe or compound animal drugs are generally not addressed by veterinary curricula. Indeed, it is not a topic easily taught. The regulations are complicated and dynamic and involve multiple role players, including regulatory (the FDA, state boards of pharmacy) and nonregulatory (United States Pharmacopeia) agencies, each of which must be consulted. The knowledge necessary to compound is equally complex and requires an understanding of basic chemistry, mathematical equations, and proper equipment and facilities. For the veterinarian sufficiently interested in compounding, finding information to guide legitimate, quality compounded products is confusing and time consuming.

Enter Dr. Lauren Forsythe's text. Her rich experience in the practice of veterinary pharmacy comes with a unique perspective of the therapeutic needs of the animal patient and the educational needs of the veterinary practitioner. She has recognized the voids and has shared her perspective through the provision of a concise, informative resource that goes a long way to filling the void. This text is the first of its kind in that it tackles both the act of veterinary compounding and the complex rules and regulations intended to minimize the risks while enhancing the benefits of safe and effective compounding of animal drugs.

Importantly, Dr. Forsythe has helped the reader to understand what constitutes a well-compounded product and how one might assess the expertise of the compounder. Assurance of the quality of a compounded preparation goes a long way to reducing the risk of adverse events, and accordingly, one chapter is dedicated to that topic. Understanding the implications of prescribing through a 503A pharmacy versus obtaining products from a 503B outsourcing facility will go a long way to helping veterinarians make the best choices for their patients.

Dr. Forsythe also provides guidance for the practice that chooses to perform their compounding in-house. A chapter addresses the physical requirements for a practice to be able to produce quality products while meeting the guidelines of the United States Pharmacopeia and the requirements of state boards of pharmacy. Equally important is support for the calculations necessary to compound. While pharmacists might be intimately familiar with the math of compounding, converting % to weight/volume, mcg to kg, and ounces to liters are tasks that are foreign to many veterinarians. Being able to reach for a one-text-does-it-all will serve the new and experienced veterinary compounder alike.

The ability to use, prescribe, or make compounded drugs is both a gift and a responsibility. Meeting the responsibility through understanding the regulations, appreciating the challenges, and accessing supportive resources is markedly facilitated by this text. This text is not intended only to the practice that currently uses compounded drugs in their patient. Rather, any practice that provides veterinary care can benefit from an understanding of the benefits of compounded medications.

Dawn Boothe

Preface

I grew up watching my parents treat everything that came to the door 24/7 for their mixed animal general practice in rural Pennsylvania. This evolved into pharmacy school and an interest in compounding. Throughout pharmacy school, clinical rotations in veterinary teaching hospitals, and a veterinary pharmacy residency, I learned that compounding is essential in many areas of veterinary practice, but it is complicated to understand the regulations, there is limited information included in most veterinary curriculums, and there is potential for unethical practices in compounding pharmacies in the name of high profits. All of this can lead to some of the high-profile compounding errors where fault is decided in court. Therefore, I found myself passionate about teaching veterinarians and veterinary students what they need to know to prescribe compounds for their patients while maximizing benefits and reducing risks. In the process of this, I learned that veterinarians have a lot of practical questions for which there is no good reference for. Therefore, the veterinarian is often left to sort through the information provided by a variety of compounding pharmacies, intermixed with an occasional CE session, and determine the validity and applicability of information that may not align.

As I spoke at conferences throughout the United States and provided webinars on basic compounding information, I frequently wished for a reference to direct people toward for further reading beyond what could be explained in a 50-minute CE. I also realized that many veterinarians are preparing at least a few compounded medications in-house but have likely not had training on techniques for ensuring that their compounds are high quality and necessary records are maintained. Understanding techniques for compounds requires a firm understanding of the regulatory, risk/benefit, and formulation development concepts. Once this information is understood, techniques can be further developed through hands on practice.

I decided if I wanted a reference for veterinary compounding written for veterinarians, then I needed to write it. This book is the product of that. I set out to explain what I thought veterinarians should know to make informed decisions about the use of compounded medications and explained the additional concepts that came up along the way. I also enlisted the help of another veterinary pharmacist that is passionate about teaching formulation development and hands-on compounding techniques to write the chapters relating to those topics. The end result is a book written for vets to answer the frequently asked questions and provide the background necessary for critically evaluating compounds that often is not feasible to provide in the limited time/word count associated with CE and editorials.

List of Acronyms

ACHC	Accreditation Commission for Health Care
AMDUCA	Animal Medicinal Drug Use Clarification Act
ANADA	Abbreviated New Animal Drug Application
API	active pharmaceutical ingredient
ASHP	American Society of Health-System Pharmacists
BOP	Board of Pharmacy
BUD	beyond-use date
CAS	Chemical Abstracts Service
cGMP	Current Good Manufacturing Practice
CNS	central nervous system
CoA	certificate of analysis
CPG	Compliance Policy Guide
CR	compounding record
CVM	Center for Veterinary Medicine
DEA	Drug Enforcement Administration
DQSA	Drug Quality and Security Act
EMP	electric mortar and pestle
EPM	equine protozoal myeloencephalitis
FD&C	Food, Drug, and Cosmetic
FDA	Food and Drug Administration
FOI	Freedom of Information
GFI	Guidance for Industry
GI	gastrointestinal tract
HPLC	high-performance liquid chromatography
IJPC	International Journal of Pharmaceutical Compounding
IM	intramuscular
IV	intravenous
LOD	loss on drying
LWQ	least weighable quantity
MFR	master formulation record
NADA	New Animal Drug Application
NDC	National Drug Code
NECC	New England Compounding Center
NF	National Formulary

NIOSH   National Institute for Occupational Safety and Health
NSAID   nonsteroidal anti-inflammatory drug
o/w   oil-in-water
PCAB   Pharmacy Compounding Accreditation Board
PIC   pharmacist in charge
QA   quality assurance
QC   quality control
QS   quantum satis
RO   reverse osmosis
SDS   safety data sheets
SOP   standard operating procedure
SQ   subcutaneous
USP   United States Pharmacopeia
UV   ultraviolet
w/o   water-in-oil

About the Companion Website

This book is accompanied by a companion website.

www.wiley.com/go/forsythe/drug

This website includes:

- Figures from the book as PowerPoint slides
- Tables from the book as PDFs

Introduction

Whether you are looking to be an informed prescriber when utilizing compounded medications or want to be able to prepare some common compounds in-house, this book is designed to provide you with the necessary information. Chapters 1–4 provide a foundation to understand the regulations at play in the veterinary compounding landscape, the risks and benefits of compounded medications, how beyond-use dates are determined, and how to select a compounding pharmacy. Chapters 5 and 6 discuss formulation development and compounding techniques for those interested in preparing common nonsterile compounds in-house. This book is written to explain what goes into answering the questions "Can this be compounded?" "Should this be compounded?" and "How do I compound this?"

In Chapter 1, the content pertaining to regulations is intentionally a more general overview. Due to the frequently changing nature and gray areas of compounding regulations, a prescriptive description of what exactly is and is not legal is not feasible to create and if created would be outdated before this book made it to print. Therefore, Chapter 1 seeks to provide background on the history of compounding regulations and review the various regulatory bodies that have an impact on compounding regulations. This information will provide you with the foundation needed to follow and interpret new regulations and critically evaluate the information surrounding them that is provided by a variety of sources.

Chapter 2 moves into the clinical considerations that accompany the regulations. The benefits of compounded medications are discussed as well as the risks. There is substantial literature supporting that the risks are prevalent in practice and not simply theoretical. Therefore, a literature review is included to provide summaries of studies looking at potency, stability, and efficacy of compounded medications prepared for both human and animal patients. The second part of this chapter will then discuss ways to decrease your risks in practice. Chapter 3 pulls out the concern about stability to provide an in-depth review of the difference between expiration and beyond-use dates and the reasoning behind how they are established. This information is then applied to understand the beyond-use variability in compounds from the same and different pharmacies.

Chapter 4 applies the information from Chapters 1–3 to evaluate a compounding pharmacy. This chapter uses two case studies of high-profile compounding errors to determine what evaluation would have been necessary to identify the quality concerns with the associated pharmacies. Following the case studies, the chapter provides detailed information about how to go about conducting an evaluation of a compounding pharmacy beyond a review of their website.

Chapters 5 and 6 assume an understanding of the information covered in Chapters 1–4 and build off that to cover formulation development considerations and compounding techniques. Chapter 5 goes through the characteristics of different types of dosage forms and the excipients that may be present. This information is then used to develop a master formulation and utilize appropriate compounding techniques in Chapter 6.

1

Compounding Regulations

A quick search of the news will provide a variety of historical cases in both human and veterinary medicine where poor-quality compounds resulted in significant morbidity and mortality. In these cases, it is often argued that something was not done legally, and if all relevant laws had been followed, the compounds would not have been made. Therefore, it behooves anyone preparing compounded medications to be well aware of the regulations surrounding compounding.

Clenbuterol Toxicosis in Three Horses in 2006 [1–3]: Three horses displayed toxicity symptoms between 12 and 24h after receiving a clenbuterol compound that contained 70-fold the amount of clenbuterol indicated on the labeling. The label indicated that the product contained 72.5 mcg/ml of clenbuterol when it actually contained 5 mg/ml. The commercial product containing clenbuterol at 72 mcg/ml had previously been used in at least one of the horses without issue. Two of the three horses were euthanized due to complications. The illegal "compounded" product was obtained from an unidentified source and administered without a prescription.

Twenty-one Polo Ponies Die Due to Compounding Error in 2009 [4, 5]: Twenty-one polo ponies competing at the US Open Polo Championship in 2009 collapsed with most dying within hours due to a selenium overdose. Franck's Pharmacy in Ocala, FL had made an error when compounding a vitamin mixture containing B-12, selenium, and other minerals, which resulted in 100 times more selenium than intended. It was determined that the horses had 10–15 times more selenium in their blood and 10–20 times more in their liver than the normal amount, which led to their deaths. The prescribed compound was intended to mimic Biodyl, which is used commonly in Europe, Asia, and Latin America. However, Biodyl is not a Food and Drug Administration (FDA)–approved product.

Fungal Meningitis Outbreak in 2012–2013 [6–8]: Three lots of a contaminated preservative-free methylprednisolone acetate injection compounded by the New England Compounding Center (NECC) in Framingham, MA were responsible for 778 fungal infections resulting in 76

Drug Compounding for Veterinary Professionals, First Edition. Lauren R. Eichstadt Forsythe and Alexandria E. Gochenauer.
© 2023 John Wiley & Sons, Inc. Published 2023 by John Wiley & Sons, Inc.
Companion Website: www.wiley.com/go/forsythe/drug

deaths across 20 states. The three lots included more than 17 000 vials of the medication which were improperly sterilized through a nonverified sterilization process and improperly tested to ensure sterility prior to being shipped throughout the United States.

Upon investigation of the compounding facility, it was noted that drugs were routinely shipped before sterility testing results were received, compounds were prepared utilizing expired ingredients, and cleaning logs were ignored as was the presence of mold and bacteria in the clean rooms. Additionally, the NECC was attempting to conceal that a technician whose license had been revoked by the Massachusetts Board of Pharmacy (BOP) was responsible for compounding sterile products.

Compounded Equine Protozoal Myeloencephalitis (EPM) Drug Linked to Equine Deaths in 2014 [9, 10]: Ten horses (eight in Florida and two in Kentucky) experienced adverse effects including seizures and fever with four horses dying after receiving a compounded EPM medication. A toltrazuril/pyrimethamine product was compounded as a paste and suspension by Wickliffe Veterinary Pharmacy of Lexington, KY containing more pyrimethamine than indicated on the labeling. Typically, the compounded paste contains 416-mg/ml toltrazuril and 17-mg/ml pyrimethamine. The lawsuit states that when the implicated product was tested, it actually contained 22 mg/ml of toltrazuril and 229 mg/ml of pyrimethamine.

Compounded EPM Drug Linked to Equine Deaths in 2019 [11, 12]: One lot of a compounded paste labeled to contain 416-mg/ml toltrazuril and 17-mg/ml pyrimethamine and compounded by Rapid Equine Solutions in Aston, PA was found to contain 18–21 times the labeled pyrimethamine concentration. The product was recalled and tested after adverse effects followed by death were noted in at least three horses. Specifically, the affected lot was found to contain 13.5 and 11.2 mg/ml of toltrazuril (3% of the labeled concentration) and 361 and 307 mg/ml of pyrimethamine (2122 and 1808% of the labeled concentration) in the two separate samples that were tested by the FDA.

However, veterinary compounding regulations are not always black and white. Common causes of confusion include the following:

- Regulations may not clearly address practical concerns.
- Human compounding regulations are often unclear whether they apply to veterinary compounding.
- Federal regulations that exempt animal patients on the federal level may be applied to animal patients at the state level.
- Compounding is largely regulated by the states resulting in significant state-to-state variation.
- Guidance for Industry (GFI) and Compliance Policy Guides (CPG) do not have the force of law but are often given significant weight.
- The regulatory landscape surrounding veterinary compounding is continuously changing and evolving to address problems and concerns that arise.
- What qualifies as compounding varies depending on which definition is being referenced.

Due to wide state-to-state variation, and regulations and standards that frequently change, this chapter is only designed to provide an overview and a starting point for further research into regulations applicable to your practice.

Organizations and Regulatory Agencies Involved with Compounding

Compounding regulations fall under a variety of agencies including:

- Food and Drug Administration
- United States Pharmacopeia (USP)
- Drug Enforcement Administration (DEA)
- State Boards of Pharmacy
- State Veterinary Boards

Food and Drug Administration

The FDA is an agency with an overall mission to "protect the public health by ensuring the safety, efficacy, and security of human and veterinary drugs, biological products, and medical devices; and by ensuring the safety of our nation's food supply, cosmetics, and products that emit radiation ..." [13]. It is further divided into nine centers, which includes the Center for Veterinary Medicine, which has a mission of "protecting human and animal health." The FDA is responsible for drug approval in the United States. Compounded drugs are not approved products, but the FDA maintains oversight through compounding regulations. However, patient-specific compounding is largely turfed to the states to regulate. Potentially, the FDA could conduct inspections, issue warning letters, and take additional actions such as injunctions, seizures, and criminal prosecution. Practically, the FDA only inspects compounding pharmacies on a "for cause" basis. Limiting factors that prevent the FDA from conducting regular inspections of compounding pharmacies include a lack of a comprehensive list of all compounding pharmacies because there is no requirement to register with the FDA, and a lack of resources to inspect the thousands of compounding pharmacies and veterinarians [14].

The FDA does complete a handful of compounding pharmacy inspections each year based on reports of adverse effects or illegal compounding. Between 2003 and 2015, the FDA conducted 39 inspections. Two reasons for warning letters issued by the FDA include large-scale compounding from bulk chemicals and compounding without a documented medical need. As a result of these inspections, multiple legal cases over the past two decades have challenged the FDA's oversight of compounded medications demonstrating that the exact role of the FDA in regulating compounded medications for nonfood animals remains unclear [14].

United States Pharmacopeia

The USP is an independent, nonprofit organization established in 1820 by a group of physicians. The physicians had noticed that ordering the same compounded medication from different apothecaries produced very different efficacy and safety. The initial intent of the USP was to standardize the quality of compounded medications. The USP evolved over the years to incorporate representatives from many different professions and to adjust to new advances such as the transition from using primarily compounded medications to manufactured medications being the predominant medication source. USP's mission statement is "To improve global health through public standards and related programs that help ensure the quality, safety, and benefit of medicines and foods" [15].

The USP is not a government agency. Instead, it operates as a standard setting body that works with FDA representatives and other government agencies. USP-NF is two compendia: the USP and the National Formulary (NF). Standards that are included in the USP-NF are based in science and developed through a transparent process that seeks stakeholder input. Active drugs that meet the USP standards are indicated with "USP" following the drug name (e.g. methimazole, USP). Compounding excipients that meet the USP standards are indicated with "NF" following the excipient name (e.g. Simple Syrup, NF). Since the USP is not a regulatory body, it does not enforce its standards. USP-NF is recognized in the Food, Drug, and Cosmetic (FD&C) Act as an official compendium, which connects USP standards with adulterating and misbranding provisions. However, the compounding standards are largely enforced by state Boards of Pharmacy. Some states incorporate USP standards into their state regulations by reference, and others may include the content with their own edits resulting in compounding regulations that vary throughout the country. While it is currently unclear and state specific whether USP standards apply to and/or are enforced for veterinarians compounding in their practices, they do clearly apply to pharmacies that compound for veterinary patients in all states.

A new version of USP-NF is published yearly with two supplements each year. The first supplement is published in February and becomes official on August 1, and the second supplement is published in June and becomes official on December 1. The content from the previous year's supplements is incorporated into each new version. The USP-NF contains chapters numbered less than 1000, which are legally enforceable, and chapters numbered greater than 1000, which are considered general information.

USP-NF provides standards for drugs (including dosage forms and compounded medications), excipients, biologics, dietary supplements, and medical devices. From the compounding aspect, there are three main chapters, USP <795> Pharmaceutical Compounding – Nonsterile Preparations, USP <797> Pharmaceutical Compounding – Sterile Preparations, and USP <800> Hazardous Drugs – Handling in Healthcare Settings. However, there are also several supporting chapters that provide additional information and requirements on topics including, but not limited to, sterility testing, quality assurance, balances and volumetric apparatus, and compounding for drug studies. USP chapters are written by expert committees made up of experts from a variety of fields relevant to the topic of the chapter. A brief summary of what each of the three main chapters mentioned above include follows. However, the exact requirements will not be discussed in this section due to their changing nature. It is expected that anyone compounding will review the relevant chapters prior to compounding and refer to them frequently.

USP Chapter <795> Pharmaceutical Compounding – Nonsterile Preparations is the chapter that outlines minimum standards for preparing nonsterile compounds. Examples of nonsterile compounds include, but are not limited to, oral liquids, topical creams, and otic medications. Topics covered include training and evaluation of those compounding, hygiene and garbing requirements, compounding facilities, cleaning and sanitizing requirements, equipment considerations, formulation considerations, compounding records and documentation, quality assurance/quality control, labeling, establishing beyond-use dates, and standard operating procedures (SOPs) as they relate to nonsterile compounding.

USP Chapter <797> Pharmaceutical Compounding – Sterile Preparations is the chapter that outlines minimum standards for preparing sterile compounds. Examples of sterile compounds include, but are not limited to, injectable medications (intramuscular, subcutaneous, and intravenous [IV]) and ophthalmic preparations. Topics covered include training and evaluation of those compounding, hygiene and garbing, compounding facilities and equipment, equipment certification and recertification, air and surface monitoring for microbiological contamination, cleaning and disinfecting, sterilization, formulation considerations, compounding documentation and records, quality assurance/quality control, labeling, beyond-use dates, and SOPs as they relate to sterile compounding.

While USP chapters <795> and <797> focus on the quality of the compound, which relates to the safety of the patient, USP Chapter <800> Hazardous Drugs – Handling in Healthcare Settings focuses on the safety of the compounder while preparing the medication. USP <800> applies to both sterile and nonsterile compounding of hazardous medications. The National Institute for Occupational Safety and Health (NIOSH) publishes a list of hazardous drugs titled NIOSH List of Antineoplastic and Other Hazardous Drugs in Healthcare Settings. This list includes different groups of hazardous drugs, and USP <800> references this list when determining if a drug is considered hazardous. However, it is important to note that USP <800> requires compounders to evaluate medications new to market since the list was last published and other drugs not considered for inclusion (i.e. veterinary-only drugs) to determine if they appear to meet the NIOSH definition of hazardous. Potential points to evaluate include drug class, drug structure, and warnings provided on the manufacturer's labeling. USP <800> includes topics such as types of exposure, responsibilities for those handling hazardous drugs, facility and engineering controls, environmental evaluations, personal protective equipment, training, hazard communication, spill control, documentation, SOPs, and handling requirements from drug receipt to administration.

Compounded Preparation Monographs present formulations used in human and/or veterinary patients. These monographs provide a specific formula including ingredients and quantities, directions to prepare the compound, a maximum beyond-use date determined by stability studies, storage and packaging information, acceptable pH ranges, and stability-indicating assays. Compounded Preparation Monographs have been included in the USP since 1820. A list of currently available monographs as well as failed studies can be found at www.usp.org. Using a compounded preparation monograph from the USP is a reliable way to make sure that a compound is being prepared in accordance with necessary stability data and formulation considerations. There are dozens of veterinary-specific monographs as well as about 200 nonveterinary specific monographs, many of which can be used for veterinary patients [16].

The USP Compounding Compendium is a collection of USP chapters and monographs that are applicable to compounding. In addition to general chapters <795>, <797>, and <800>, the Compounding Compendium includes the following general chapters:

– <825> Radiopharmaceuticals – Preparation, Compounding, Dispensing, and Repackaging
– <1160> Pharmaceutical Calculations in Prescription Compounding
– <1163> Quality Assurance in Pharmaceutical Compounding
– <1168> Compounding for Phase I Investigational Studies
– <1176> Prescription Balances and Volumetric Apparatus

The Compendium also includes the supporting general chapters that are referenced in the compounding-specific chapters listed above.

Drug Enforcement Administration

The DEA's mission is "to enforce the controlled substance laws and regulations of the United States and bring to the criminal and civil justice system of the United States, or any other competent jurisdiction, those organizations and principal members of organizations, involved in the growing, manufacture, or distribution of controlled substances appearing in or destined for illicit traffic in the United States; and to recommend and support nonenforcement programs aimed at reducing the availability of illicit controlled substances on the domestic and international markets" [17]. Based on this mission, the DEA is concerned with compounding that involves controlled substances, but they are not involved in compounding of noncontrolled substances. Practically,

DEA compliance with regards to compounding involves following all controlled substance regulations when preparing compounded medications utilizing controlled substances.

State Boards of Pharmacy

State Boards of Pharmacy are responsible for overseeing the practice of pharmacy within their state, which includes compounding done by those licensed under the BOP such as pharmacists and pharmacy technicians. Pharmacy boards also require out-of-state pharmacies to be licensed for each state they are shipping to. This allows the pharmacy board to hold out-of-state pharmacies to the same standards as those located within the state. This becomes significant with compounded medications because states may have vastly different requirements for compounding pharmacies with regard to licensure and inspection. Depending on the way a state is set up, the pharmacy board may have oversight of all drug dispensing regardless of profession. Therefore, in some states, the pharmacy board has oversight of medication-related professional activities that veterinarians are engaged in which would include compounding.

The amount of oversight and available data from each state varies greatly. One example of a state program is the Missouri BOP. In 2003, the Missouri BOP started a program that tests a sample of compounded products each year of several different drug types and dosage forms. In 2020, the board tested 57 compounds for potency and, if applicable, sterility and endotoxins. The dosage forms tested include capsules, IV solutions, inhalation solutions, injectables, oral suspensions, tablets, topical creams/ointments, and topical solutions. Of the 57 compounds tested, 11 (19.3%) compounds representing 10 different active ingredients had unsatisfactory results due to potency being outside of the allowed ±10% or USP stated range [18].

The National Association of Boards of Pharmacy provides contact information and websites for each state pharmacy board at https://nabp.pharmacy/about/boards-of-pharmacy.

State Veterinary Boards

State veterinary boards are responsible for overseeing the practice of veterinary medicine within their state. Since veterinarians are legally allowed to compound medications for their patients, veterinary boards would oversee this. However, not all states have compounding laws written into their veterinary practice act, which can make this a gray area.

The American Association of Veterinary State Boards provides contact information and websites for each state veterinary board at https://www.aavsb.org/public-resources/find-regulatory-board-information.

Compliance Policy Guides and Guidance for Industry Documents

Other important concepts to define are CPGs and GFIs. The FDA issues CPGs and GFIs when it determines something is illegal but necessary under certain circumstances or they determine that a topic requires additional clarification. These documents indicate the FDA's current regulatory priorities and are subject to modification and withdrawal. They do not have the force of law. However, they are often the best indicator available of how the FDA intends to enforce various regulations and may be used by states to guide their compounding regulations. While CPGs and GFIs appear similar, they are written for different audiences. CPGs are written to guide inspectors on what to look for during inspections, while GFIs are written to guide the industry on compliance.

For practical purposes, both types of documents provide insight into the FDA's current thought process and should be used to guide compliance with the regulations.

CPGs and GFIs are used when the FDA plans to exercise its regulatory discretion. The following is a daily life example of this concept.

> In a specific area, the speed limit is 50 miles per hour (mph). However, the local police department has decided that they will only pull someone over for speeding if they are going faster than 60 mph. Since the speed limit is 50 mph, it is illegal to go faster than that. However, the police department is exercising its regulatory discretion by choosing not to enforce the speed limit unless someone is exceeding it by more than 10 mph.

What Is Compounding?

The exact definition of compounding varies depending on whether the FDA or the USP definition is being referenced. The FDA defines compounding as, "the process of combining, mixing or altering ingredients to create a medication tailored to the needs of an individual patient. Compounding includes the combining of two or more drugs. Compounded drugs are not FDA approved" [19]. In Section 503a of the FD&C Act, which applies to patient-specific compounding, the FDA states, "as used in this section, the term 'compounding' does not include mixing, reconstituting, or other such acts that are performed in accordance with directions contained in approved labeling provided by the product's manufacturer and other manufacturer directions consistent with that labeling" [19].

Historically, the USP defined compounding as, "The preparation, mixing, assembling, altering, packaging, and labeling of a drug, drug-delivery device, or device in accordance with a licensed practitioner's prescription, medication order, or initiative based on the practitioner/patient/pharmacist/compounder relationship in the course of professional practice" [20]. However, with the 2022 revisions, the nonsterile compounding definition was updated to, "combining, admixing, diluting, pooling, reconstituting other than as provided in the manufacturer's labeling, or other altering a drug product or bulk drug substance to create a nonsterile preparation." The updated Chapter <795> goes on to state that the following are not considered compounding:

- Reconstitution of a conventionally manufactured nonsterile product in accordance with the directions contained in the manufacturer approved labeling
- Repackaging of conventionally manufactured drug products
- Breaking or cutting a tablet into smaller portions
- Preparation of a single dose for a single patient when administration will begin within 4 h [21]

These updates bring the USP and FDA definitions in line with regard to what is and is not considered compounding. Table 1.1 shows the difference in compounding definitions between the two USP versions and the FDA version. It should be noted that other groups such as AVMA have provided definitions of compounding, and these may vary from the USP and FDA definitions.

In contrast, manufacturing is defined as, "The production, preparation, propagation, conversion or processing of a drug or device, either directly or indirectly, by extraction from substances of natural origin or independently by means of chemical or biological synthesis and includes any packaging or repackaging the substance(s) or the labeling or re-labeling of its

Table 1.1 Examples of compounding based on the FDA and USP definitions.

Example	Compounding under the FDA definition	Compounding under the old USP definition	Compounding under the new (2022) USP definition	Notes
Reconstituting Clavamox (amoxicillin/ clavulanate) powder for suspension with 14 ml of water to a final concentration of 62.5 mg/ml with a 10-d beyond-use date when stored in the fridge **which is in accordance with the manufacturer's labeling**.	No	Yes	No	This is an example of preparing a medication based on the manufacturer's labeling.
Reconstituting doxycycline powder with **25 ml** of water to make a **10-mg/ml** suspension that can be stored at room temperature for 2 wk when the manufacturer labeling indicates using **50 ml** of water for a **5-mg/ml** suspension.	Yes	Yes	Yes	This is another example of reconstituting an antibiotic, but there are changes from what the manufacturer's labeling indicates. By adjusting the final concentration of the product, it now falls under compounding based on the FDA definition in addition to the USP definition.
Crushing 250-mg metronidazole tablets and mixing with water to make a 50-mg/ml oral suspension.	Yes	Yes	Yes	This is manipulating a commercial product in a way different than the approved labeling.
Drawing up a ketamine bolus dose to be given immediately.	No	No	No	This is preparing a drug for immediate administration.

container and the promotion and marketing of such drugs or devices. Manufacturing also includes any preparation of a drug or device that is sold for resale by pharmacies, practitioners, or other persons [22]."

The main difference between the compounding and manufacturing definitions is that compounding is designed to be patient-specific and based on a practitioner's order or prescription, and manufacturing is not. Therefore, traditional compounding should not look like manufacturing. However, there are instances where compounds are needed on a large scale and/or on hand in a practice for immediate use. In these cases, the amount of dosage units being prescribed and the fact that they may be kept on hand in a practice causes their preparation to look a lot like manufacturing. That is where the Drug Quality and Security Act (DQSA) comes into play by defining the requirements for preparing large quantities of compounded products. A future section will discuss how this act affects compounded medications for veterinary patients.

The Food, Drug, and Cosmetic Act

The FD&C Act that was originally passed in 1938 became the first piece of legislation to require that drugs be proven safe. In 1968, the act was amended to include veterinary medications with the intention of requiring them to be safe, effective, and not leave residues in the human food supply. At that point, it became unsafe and, therefore, illegal to utilize medications in any way other than what the FDA-approved labeling indicated. Therefore, medications had to be used within the following constraints:

– An FDA-approved drug labeled for use in animals
– Used in the species (and any additional qualifiers such as age, reproductive status, etc.) for which it is labeled
– For the labeled indication
– At the dose and frequency indicated on the label
– For the labeled duration

These restrictions were impossible to comply with in veterinary medicine. However, the FDA acknowledged that there were instances when extra-label use is necessary in veterinary medicine. Therefore, they issued two CPGs: "Extra-Label Use of New Animal Drugs in Food-Producing Animals" that addressed food animals and "Human-Labeled Drugs Distributed and Used in Animal Medicine" that addressed nonfood animals. Eventually, these were given the force of law as the Animal Medicinal Drug Use Clarification Act (AMDUCA).

Animal Medicinal Drug Use Clarification Act

The AMDUCA is a pivotal piece of legislation from 1994 which legalized extra-label drug use (ELDU) with certain restrictions. The AMDUCA divided patients into food animals and nonfood animals based on intended use and described when off-label use would be appropriate for each group.

The following outlines when ELDU is legal in each group. It is important to note that it is required for a valid veterinarian, client, patient relationship to be in place prior to any ELDU.

Nonfood animals

1) The first product choice should be a veterinary-approved product used as labeled or extra-label use of a human-approved drug according to the labeled veterinary dose.
2) When a product cannot be used as labeled, a veterinary-approved product or human-approved product can be used in an extra-label manner.
3) If there is no approved product that can be used as labeled or extra-label, then a compounded product can be used. When utilizing a compounded medication, it is important that there is a clinical justification. Compounding a mimic product is only acceptable when the approved product is not available. Compounding a mimic for economic reasons is not legal [23]. Valid reasons for compounding include the following:
   a) Dose: When the commercial product cannot be used to administer the appropriate dose. For example, piroxicam is available as a human product in 10- and 20-mg capsules. However, at a dose of 0.3 mg/kg in dogs, many patients require a smaller dosage than 10 mg.
   b) Dosage form: Patients may require a liquid medication when the only approved products are tablets.

    c) Compliance issues: When patients are difficult to medicate, this can lead to decreased compliance which decreases drug efficacy and can lead to resistance in the case of antibiotics or disease exacerbation. Compounds can be utilized to provide a flavor and/or dosage form that is more readily accepted by the patient such as a flavored liquid or a chewable treat.

    d) Avoidance of allergens/toxic ingredients: When patients are allergic to an inactive ingredient or the commercial product contains a toxic inactive ingredient, compounds can be utilized to provide a version of the medication that the patient can tolerate.

Food animals: In addition to the guidelines below, there are certain drugs and drug classes that are banned from extra-label use in food animals.

1) The first choice should be to use a veterinary-approved product according to the label. This includes observing the stated withholding and/or slaughter withdrawal times.

2) If a product cannot be used as labeled, the extra-label use of a veterinary-approved product labeled for use in food animals is the next option. By using a product labeled for food animals, it provides a starting point for determining an appropriate withdrawal/withholding time.

3) If a food animal product cannot be used, the extra-label use of a veterinary-approved, nonfood animal drug or a human-approved medication can be considered. This is only acceptable if a withdrawal/withholding time can be determined in collaboration with FARAD.

4) The last resort is use of a compounded product made from an approved veterinary or human drug.

Since compounding for food animals should only be done as a last resort, the remainder of this text will focus on nonfood animals.

Preparing Compounds from an Approved Product or a Pure Drug Powder

From a compounding perspective, AMDUCA and ELDU are important because compounded medications are not FDA approved, which means they were not legal prior to AMDUCA either. The AMDUCA mentions compounded medications 11 times, but only defines them as being created by modifying an FDA-approved product. This means that AMDUCA legalized creating a suspension by crushing commercially available tablets but did not legalize preparing the same suspension from pure drug powder. Pure drug powder may also be referred to as bulk chemical or active pharmaceutical ingredient.

While some compounded medications can be prepared by manipulating a commercially available product, there are several instances where this may not be feasible or appropriate. A few examples of this are as follows:

– The commercially available product is on backorder: If the reason for compounding is because the commercial product cannot be obtained, the commercial product cannot be used to prepare the compound necessitating the use of bulk chemical.

– There is no approved product with that active ingredient: Historically, this was the case for potassium bromide, which was widely used, but not FDA approved until 2021. Another example is cisapride, which was FDA approved as a human medication at one point but was then pulled from the market in 2000 [24].

– The approved product is not feasible to use: This is the case when the only approved product is a chewable tablet, which will not make a high-quality compound due to the inactive ingredients. This can also occur with some coated tablets. Another example would be: if a liquid commercial

product is too dilute for practical administration, it is not practical to use as the drug source for making a more concentrated product.
– The patient has an allergy or intolerance to an inactive ingredient in the approved product: In this case, the purpose of compounding is often to avoid the ingredient the patient is allergic to or cannot tolerate. Therefore, the commercial product cannot be used.

While the above examples illustrate why it is not always possible to create a compound by manipulating the FDA-approved product, that does not change the fact that the AMDUCA did not legalize it. Since the AMDUCA was passed, there have been several versions of CPGs and GFIs that attempted to address compounding from bulk chemicals. However, at the time of writing, there is no clear regulation, and the topic remains controversial and changes frequently. The reader is advised to consult current state and federal regulations to determine legality of using bulk chemicals to compound.

Federal Versus State Law [8]

Patient-specific compounding is under the jurisdiction of the states like most other licensed health care activities. In contrast, human office use compounding is under the jurisdiction of the FDA. However, this was not always clearly defined as multiple judicial cases in the early 2000s led to confusion about which compounding practices were under federal versus state oversight. At the time of writing, where veterinary office use compounding falls is unclear. This means that federal compounding regulations are limited and often big picture, and exact details of compounding are left to each state to determine. Practically, most of these state compounding regulations are enforced by each state's BOP since the majority of compounding is performed by pharmacists. However, state veterinary boards may choose to include compounding topics in their practice act as well, which would apply to veterinarians preparing compounded medications in their practices.

It is important to be aware of what your state's compounding regulations are and determine how to comply. It is recommended to consult both the veterinary practice act and the pharmacy practice act in your state. When federal and state laws differ, the stricter law must be followed. It also varies by state whether the pharmacy board has any oversight of veterinarians preparing compounded medications. Therefore, it is advisable to determine which regulatory agencies oversee drugs in veterinary practice in your state. Regardless, it is good practice to be aware of and comply with state pharmacy compounding regulations. These regulations are designed to ensure high-quality compounds for both humans and animals making them applicable to veterinarians as well even if not enforceable.

One caveat to consider when looking at state regulations is how they incorporate USP standards. Some states do not incorporate USP at all and instead write their own compounding standards into their practice acts. These standards are similar to, but often not identical to the USP standards. However, other states reference USP by stating that they require compliance with USP chapters 795 and 797. For states that have their regulations written this way, the compounding requirements are subject to change whenever USP publishes chapter revisions. While major revisions are infrequent and involve significant stakeholder input, it is important to be aware of the changes if you are in a state that incorporates USP into state regulations by reference.

Another area of state oversight to consider is that states require pharmacies shipping medications into the state to be licensed with that state. Therefore, if a prescription is placed with a pharmacy in Pennsylvania and they will be shipping it to a clinic or patient in Maryland, the pharmacy also needs to be licensed in Maryland. For some states, licensure requires that the out-of-state pharmacy follow the same regulations as in-state pharmacies, but how this is enforced varies widely. Other states only require the pharmacy to meet the requirements in the state in which they are physically located, and a few states require the pharmacy to comply with the compounding regulations in both the state where they are located as well as the state granting the license. Still additional states may compare their state regulations to the regulations of the state where the pharmacy is located and determine if they are comparable and then determine compliance requirements. To further complicate matters, what each state does is subject to change. For enforcement, most states have some type of inspection requirement for out-of-state pharmacies that are shipping sterile compounds into the state, and these requirements may or may not align with the in-state pharmacy inspection requirements. The requirements range from no specified frequency to required yearly inspections. Nonsterile compounding pharmacies may or may not be subjected to the same inspection requirements as sterile compounding pharmacies. Best practice is that out-of-state pharmacies are inspected at the same frequency as in-state pharmacies, but this is not necessarily the case. While a few states will inspect out-of-state pharmacies or identify acceptable third parties to complete the required inspections, many states rely on the regulatory agency where the pharmacy is located to conduct the inspections as they may not have the legal authority to conduct inspections of pharmacies located out of state.

Office Use Compounding

Compounding is intended to be the preparation of a unique medication to meet the needs of an individual patient. Therefore, it stands to reason that compounded medications should have the individual patient identified by way of a prescription prior to preparing the compound. In fact, that concept is included in both the FDA and USP definitions of compounding. However, sometimes compounded medications are needed urgently. Therapy cannot be delayed while waiting for the compounded medication to be prepared, especially if the medication is being prepared by another location and will require shipping. In those cases, it is necessary to have a compounded medication prepared and on hand for use in the office in anticipation of a patient needing it. This is the reasoning for office use compounding. Office use compounding is the process of having medication on hand that was not compounded for a specific patient to meet these needs [25]. Examples where office use compounds may be necessary include the following:

– Metronidazole 50-mg capsules for starting immediate treatment in a patient that is too small to dose with the 250-mg human tablets
– Diluted ephedrine for emergency administration to small animal patients
– Diluted acepromazine for use in small patients
– Enrofloxacin suspension for a patient that is not able to be dosed with the tablet or injectable formulations
– CaEDTA for use in raptors with lead poisoning

While there is clearly a need for office use compounds, there are additional risks when utilizing compounds that are not prepared for a specific patient. Traditional compounded medications are not required to be tested to prove that they are stable and contain what they are labeled to contain. When compounding, many ingredients look similar, making it possible to accidentally select the wrong ingredient. While there are checks in place to avoid this error, human error is still possible. When compounding for an individual patient, if an error occurs, it only reaches that one patient.

However, if an error occurs when preparing a batch for office use, that medication may be distributed to several patients, making the impact of an error more significant. Therefore, office use compounding needs must be weighed against the potential risk for a risk–benefit analysis. For this reason, regulations at both the state and federal levels address office use compounding. At the federal level, there is the DQSA. State regulations regarding office use interpret and/or further define acceptable office use in conjunction with the DQSA.

Drug Quality and Security Act [26]

Office use compounding was historically regulated by the states. However, after the meningitis outbreak in 2012–2013, the FDA decided that there needed to be federal oversight for large volume compounding facilities that are distributing sterile products throughout the country. The result is the DQSA, which splits compounding pharmacies into two groups. These are 503a or traditional compounding pharmacies and 503b or outsourcing facilities. Pharmacies licensed as 503a pharmacies compound in the traditional sense where they make patient-specific medications pursuant to a prescription. In contrast, those licensed as 503b outsourcing facilities are manufacturing compounded medications. These outsourcing facilities were the FDA's answer to regulating sterile compounds being distributed throughout the country for office use. As such, outsourcing facilities are overseen by the FDA, in addition to the state boards, and they need to prepare sterile compounds. Because these facilities must comply with manufacturing standards, small, patient-specific batches are not practical. To meet the needs of unique patients, traditional compounding pharmacies prepare small batches of unique medications.

At the federal level, the DQSA indicates that office use compounds must be prepared by a 503b outsourcing facility. However, the DQSA does not apply to preparing compounds for veterinary patients, and there is not any similar law that does apply to veterinary patients. This puts the legality of office use compounding for veterinary patients back at the state level. However, there are still multiple gray areas surrounding office use in several states:

- Some states indicate that office use compounding is not allowed by 503a pharmacies and do not differentiate between veterinary and human office use compounding.
- Some states have office use regulations that align with the DQSA for human compounding and have different regulations for veterinary compounding. This can lead to confusion at the individual compounding pharmacy level when they prepare compounds for both humans and animals. These regulations vary based on how states evaluate the risk–benefit ratio. For example, some may determine that benefit outweighs risk when administering the medication in hospital and dispensing enough to treat the patient while waiting for a compounding pharmacy to prepare and ship the medication based on a patient-specific prescription. After that initial time frame, the risk may outweigh the benefit since a patient-specific prescription could have been obtained.

Finding Additional Information

Due to the ever-changing nature of compounding regulations, and the wide state-to-state variability, this chapter does not go into detail about exactly what the regulations require. However, the following references shown in Table 1.2 are where you can find more information on current regulations.

Table 1.2 References for information on current compounding regulations.

Reference	Link	Information available
USP Website	http://www.usp.org	– Background information on USP – Current expert committee members – Updates on chapter updates in progress and key dates for comment submission – USP publications available for purchase
USP Compounding Compendia	Purchase at https://www.usp.org/products/usp-compounding-compendium	– Compounding chapters – Compounded Preparation Monographs
State Pharmacy Boards	List of all websites found at: https://nabp.pharmacy/about/boards-of-pharmacy	– State regulations
State Veterinary Boards	List of all websites found at: https://www.aavsb.org/public-resources/find-regulatory-board-information	– State regulations
AVMA	http://www.avma.org	– News and position statements on compounding legislation – Summary of state office use laws – AMDUCA ELDU requirements
FDA	http://www.fda.gov	– GFIs and CPGs – Warning letters issued to compounding pharmacies – Current and resolved drug shortages – New drug approvals – Approved animal drugs and marketing status – Approved human drugs and marketing status – Appropriate drug disposal – Indexed drugs for Minor Use/Minor Species – Adverse event reporting – Compounding risk alerts
DailyMed	https://dailymed.nlm.nih.gov/dailymed	– Package inserts for FDA-approved human and veterinary medications. **Note:** package inserts differ depending on the manufacturer.
AMDUCA	https://www.ecfr.gov/cgi-bin/text-idx?SID=054808d261de27898e02fb175b7c9ff9&node=21:6.0.1.1.16&rgn=div5	– ELDU requirements

Table 1.2 (Continued)

Reference	Link	Information available
DQSA	https://www.fda.gov/drugs/human-drug-compounding/text-compounding-quality-act	– 503a pharmacies versus 503b outsourcing facilities
cGMP	https://www.accessdata.fda.gov/scripts/cdrh/cfdocs/cfcfr/CFRSearch.cfm?CFRPart=211	– Requirements for medications prepared by 503b outsourcing facilities and for manufacturing approved medications

References

1 Schultz, K. (2006). Counterfeit clenbuterol found in treated horses. https://www.dvm360.com/view/counterfeit-clenbuterol-found-treated-horses (accessed 25 December 2022).

2 (2006). Horse deaths associated with unapproved drug. American Veterinary Medical Association. https://www.avma.org/javma-news/2007-01-01/horse-deaths-associated-unapproved-drug (accessed 25 December 2022).

3 Thompson, J.A., Mirza, M.H., Barker, S.A. et al. (2011). Clenbuterol toxicosis in three Quarter Horse racehorses after administration of a compounded product. *J. Am. Vet. Med. Assoc.* 239 (6): 842–849. https://doi.org/10.2460/JAVMA.239.6.842.

4 Crisco, A. (2016). $2.5M verdict slaps compounding lab and pharmacist in trial over poisoning deaths of 21 polo ponies. https://blog.cvn.com/2.5m-verdict-slaps-compounding-lab-and-pharmacist-in-trial-over-poisoning-deaths-of-21-polo-ponies (accessed 25 December 2022).

5 Osborne, M. (2009). Compounding issues resurface in wake of ponies' deaths. American Veterinary Medical Association. https://www.avma.org/javma-news/2009-06-15/compounding-issues-resurface-wake-ponies-deaths (accessed 25 December 2022).

6 (2019). January 31, 2018: New England Compounding Center pharmacist sentenced for role in nationwide fungal meningitis outbreak. FDA. https://www.fda.gov/inspections-compliance-enforcement-and-criminal-investigations/press-releases/january-31-2018-new-england-compounding-center-pharmacist-sentenced-role-nationwide-fungal (accessed 25 December 2022).

7 (2015). Multistate outbreak of fungal meningitis and other infections. HAI | CDC. https://www.cdc.gov/hai/outbreaks/meningitis.html (accessed 25 December 2022).

8 (2018). State oversight of drug compounding. The Pew Charitable Trusts. https://www.pewtrusts.org/en/research-and-analysis/reports/2018/02/state-oversight-of-drug-compounding (accessed 25 December 2022).

9 Equimanagement. (2015). Medicine C for V. CVM updates – FDA alerts horse owners and veterinarians about adverse events associated with certain unapproved compounded drugs in horses.

10 Angst, F. (2014). Horse owners file lawsuits against Wickliffe. BloodHorse. https://www.bloodhorse.com/horse-racing/articles/113691/horse-owners-file-lawsuits-against-wickliffe (accessed 25 December 2022).

11 (2020). Rapid Equine Solutions, LLC - 595556 - 06/12/2020. FDA. https://www.fda.gov/inspections-compliance-enforcement-and-criminal-investigations/warning-letters/rapid-equine-solutions-llc-595556-06122020 (accessed 25 December 2022).

12 (2019). Compounded unapproved animal drugs from rapid equine solutions linked to three horse deaths.FDA.https://www.fda.gov/animal-veterinary/cvm-updates/compounded-unapproved-animal-drugs-rapid-equine-solutions-linked-three-horse-deaths (accessed 25 December 2022).

13 (2018). What we do. FDA. https://www.fda.gov/about-fda/what-we-do (accessed 25 December 2022).

14 Drug Compounding for Animals FDA Could Improve Oversight with Better Information and Guidance Report to Congressional Committees United States Government Accountability Office. (2015).

15 The history of medicine quality. https://www.usp.org/200-anniversary/history-of-medicine-quality (accessed 25 December 2022).

16 Compounded preparations monographs (CPMs). USP. https://www.usp.org/compounding/compounded-preparation-monographs (accessed 25 December 2022).

17 Mission. https://www.dea.gov/about/mission (accessed 25 December 2022).

18 Parson, M.L., Lindley-Myers, C., and Ledgerwood, S. (2021). Annual Report Annual Report FY 2020 Missouri Board of Pharmacy. www.pr.mo.gov/pharmacists (accessed 29 May 2021).

19 (2022). Compounding and the FDA: questions and answers. FDA. https://www.fda.gov/drugs/human-drug-compounding/compounding-and-fda-questions-and-answers#what (accessed 25 December 2022).

20 ASHP. Compounding frequently asked questions 1. Where can I find the compounding guidances? https://www.google.com/url?sa=t&rct=j&q=&esrc=s&source=web&cd=&ved=2ahUKEwjlvqDc48r9AhVEjIkEHRjxBRwQFnoECA0QAw&url=https%3A%2F%2Fwww.ashp.org%2F-%2Fmedia%2Fassets%2Fadvocacy-issues%2Fdocs%2Fcompounding-guidances-frequently-asked-questions.pdf&usg=AOvVaw0JXKvEkIbAoyUruea1MCmO (accessed 29 May 2021).

21 United States Pharmacopeial Convention (2022). USP general chapter <795> pharmaceutical compounding – nonsterile preparations (2022 update). *Compounding Compendium*. Frederick, MD: USP.

22 Wyoming Administrative Code | State Regulations | US Law. LII/Legal Information Institute. https://www.law.cornell.edu/regulations/wyoming/Pharmacy-Board-of-Pharmacy-Board-of-Ch-13-SS-2 (accessed 25 December 2022).

23 Compounding FAQ for veterinarians. American Veterinary Medical Association. https://www.avma.org/resources-tools/animal-health-and-welfare/animal-health/compounding/compounding-faq-veterinarians (accessed 25 December 2022).

24 Drugs@FDA: FDA-approved drugs. https://www.accessdata.fda.gov/scripts/cder/daf/index.cfm?event=overview.process&ApplNo=020210 (accessed 25 December 2022).

25 FDA, CDER (2016). Prescription requirement under section 503A of the Federal Food, Drug, and Cosmetic Act guidance for industry. http://www.fda.gov/Drugs/GuidanceComplianceRegulatoryInformation/Guidances/default.htm (accessed 29 May 2021).

26 (2020). Compounding laws and policies. FDA. https://www.fda.gov/drugs/human-drug-compounding/compounding-laws-and-policies (accessed 25 December 2022).

2

Risk–Benefit Analysis of Compounded Medications

Benefits of Compounded Products

Compounded medications provide several benefits when used in veterinary medicine with these benefits often being species and patient specific. In general, these benefits fall into five different categories: dosage form, dosage strength, flavoring, eliminating ingredients, and availability. This section will discuss each of these categories in more detail. It is important to note that cost is not listed as a potential benefit. As discussed in Chapter 1, compounding for the benefit that it is less expensive than using a commercially available dosage form is not legal [1].

Dosage Form

With the wide variety of species and size variation within many of these species, it is not practical to expect that Food and Drug Administration (FDA)-approved products will be available in the appropriate dosage form for every patient. Many approved products may only be available as a tablet or capsule, which can be difficult to administer to ferrets and birds. There may also be specific patient and caregiver preferences regarding which dosage form (and route of administration) is easiest to administer. In addition to ease of administration, dosage form can also be used for ease of dosing. For example, if you have a patient that needs a medication that is likely to be titrated over time, a liquid can be great because it allows simply adjusting the volume administered when the dosage needs changed versus a solid dosage form where you are more limited in the ability to make small dose adjustments. For example, being able to reliably adjust a dose by 25% based on therapeutic drug monitoring will likely be easier to achieve compliance if you can direct the client to administer a different volume of liquid versus prescribing a new tablet strength.

Dosage forms are closely tied to the route of administration. For each route of administration (oral, transdermal, topical, subcutaneous, etc.), there are several dosage forms that could be employed. When determining which dosage form to utilize, the first step is to determine what route of administration is ideal. The route of administration can also be used to decrease the incidence of adverse effects. One study found that transdermal methimazole had a 20% lower incidence of gastrointestinal adverse effects compared to oral administration [2]. If a nontraditional route of administration, like transdermal, is desired, it is a good idea to have a second choice determined in case that the route is not feasible with the specific medication or species. Table 2.1 lists routes of administration and dosage form options for that route as well as pros and cons of that route of administration. More details can be found in Chapter 5.

Drug Compounding for Veterinary Professionals, First Edition. Lauren R. Eichstadt Forsythe and Alexandria E. Gochenauer.
© 2023 John Wiley & Sons, Inc. Published 2023 by John Wiley & Sons, Inc.
Companion Website: www.wiley.com/go/forsythe/drug

Table 2.1 Pros and cons of administration routes.

Route of administration	Pros and cons of this route	Common dosage forms used
Oral	Pros: – Nonsterile – Can be flavored to ease administration – Dosage is typically well-defined – Inexpensive to prepare – Readily available at most compounding pharmacies Cons: – Administration can be challenging – Often slower acting than parenteral routes – Systemic side effects	Tablets, capsules, treats, solutions, suspensions, emulsions, pastes, syrups, powders
Transdermal (systemic)	Pros: – Nonsterile – Easy to administer – Readily available at most compounding pharmacies – Systemic effects with potential for less GI side effects compared to oral Cons: – Appropriate dosage often not well-defined and available data mostly limited to feline patients – Increased risk of caregiver drug absorption – Topical irritation commonly occurs – Limited surface area results in dosage limitations – Often slower acting than parenteral routes – Systemic side effects may occur	Gels, ointments, creams
Topical (skin; nonsystemic)	Pros: – Nonsterile – Easy to administer – Readily available at most compounding pharmacies – Avoids systemic adverse effects Cons: – May be groomed off (other than shampoos) – Effects limited to application site – Increased risk of caregiver drug absorption – Topical irritation may occur	Solutions, ointments, shampoos, mousses, creams, gels
Otic	Pros: – Nonsterile – Easy to administer – Readily available at most compounding pharmacies – Avoids systemic adverse effects Cons: – Often stability is unknown	Solutions, suspensions, ointments
Rectal	Pros: – Nonsterile – Readily available at most compounding pharmacies – Absorbed quickly – Can usually be administered easily Cons: – Caregivers may object to administration	Solutions

Table 2.1 (Continued)

Route of administration	Pros and cons of this route	Common dosage forms used
Intranasal	Pros: – Nonsterile (when not inhaled) – Readily available at most compounding pharmacies – Absorbed quickly – Can usually be administered easily with training Cons: May require an atomizer syringe attachment for administration	Solutions
Intravenous	Pros: – Full dose is bioavailable – Dosage is often well-defined Cons: – Additional skillset needed for administration and may not be feasible for clients to administer in some species – Requires sterility – Only available at pharmacies that have sterile compounding facilities	Solutions
Intramuscular	Pros: – Generally, well absorbed in short timeframe – Dosage is often well-defined Cons: – Additional skillset needed for administration and may not be feasible for clients to administer in some species – Requires sterility – Only available at pharmacies that have sterile compounding facilities	Solutions, suspensions
Subcutaneous	Pros: Generally, well absorbed in short timeframe – Dosage is often well-defined – Clients can usually be trained to administer in species where this route is commonly used Cons: – Requires sterility – Only available at pharmacies that have sterile compounding facilities	Solutions, suspensions
Ophthalmic	Pros: – Easy to administer – Avoids systemic adverse effects Cons: – Requires sterility – Only available at pharmacies that have sterile compounding facilities – Limited tear film volume in the eye requires separation of different drugs – Irritation may occur	Solutions, suspensions, ointments

Flavoring

Along with dosage form considerations, the addition of flavoring can be helpful to facilitate compliance. A wide variety of flavors can be added to oral medications to create an enticing smell and/or an acceptable taste for a patient. Bitterness suppressor can be added to help counteract the bitterness of a medication. It is important to note that when selecting flavoring, if a sweet flavor is desired, a sweetener will also be required as flavoring and sweetening are two separate processes. Sweet and bitter are antagonistic tastes; therefore, sweetener can be added to counteract bitter medications. This appears to work in species that are thought to lack the ability to taste sweet flavors like cats [3]. When determining which flavor to select, a good rule of thumb is to ask the caregiver what flavor their animal is likely to prefer, but sometimes it is not necessary to pick the animal's favorite flavor but rather to make the flavor as nonoffensive as possible. For cats, sweet flavors may still be used because they can be helpful for creating a nonoffensive flavor by reducing the bitterness and foul taste. Flavors like marshmallow and vanilla butternut are commonly used for this purpose. If trying to identify a desirable flavor, there are assumptions that can be made based on species such as meat for dogs, fish for cats, and apple for horses. However, caregivers often know their specific animal best and can provide a more tailored recommendation. For example, butterscotch may be an ideal flavor for a particular horse despite not being something typically expected for that species.

Flavoring options are available from a variety of sources and can fall into three main types: powder, liquid, and homemade. Powder flavors are compatible with either aqueous or oil-based liquids as well as solid dosage forms like treats. Liquid flavors may be either oil-based or aqueous, and it is important that the appropriately formulated flavor is used based on the formulation it is being added to. Homemade flavors are those that are made in-house versus manufactured. An example of this would be blending multiple types of fish to create a "triple fish" flavor. The use of homemade flavors can greatly increase acceptance, but they come with inherent risks due to the lack of preservatives and other excipients found in commercially available flavors. Due to these uncertainties, addition of flavor to a commercial product falls into the realm of compounding as flavoring can affect the stability of the drug. An in-depth review of flavoring options and important considerations when adding them to formulations can be found in Chapter 5.

Dosage Strength

The same species and size variety mentioned above also create a need for dosage strengths that are not commercially available. When compounding for the purpose of creating a new dosage strength, it is important to ensure that there is a clinical difference between the compound and the commercially available option. There is not a specified number of milligrams difference that is required to be clinically different nor is it practical to create one. What constitutes a clinical difference varies depending on the drug and the patient. What is important to keep in mind is the accuracy of compounded and commercial products. Every medication has an allowed margin of error in which it is still considered acceptable. For manufactured products, this margin of error is specified by United States Pharmacopeia (USP) for specific drugs. For compounded products, the USP-allowed margin of error is ±10% [4]. Therefore, a compounded capsule labeled to contain 100 mg of drug may legally contain anywhere from 90 to 110 mg of that drug and be considered acceptable. For manufactured products, it is best to determine the range for a specific drug. However, if that is not feasible, ±10% is a common assumption [4].

Let us look at the following example: Piroxicam is a nonsteroidal anti-inflammatory drug (NSAID) utilized to treat transitional cell carcinoma in dogs. It is well documented that the optimal dose is 0.3 mg/kg [5]. It is also known that NSAIDs have a risk of causing severe adverse effects in dogs when overdosed. Therefore, this medication has a narrow therapeutic index, making it critical to utilize a product providing the optimal dose based on patient size. Piroxicam is commercially available as an FDA-approved human medication in 10- and 20-mg capsules. While these are acceptable to utilize in dogs needing one of those dosages, the fact that they are capsules and the relatively high strength make them impractical to accurately dose many patients. Therefore, a compounded product is often utilized. When determining what strengths are appropriate to compound, we would want to take the commercial strength and add or subtract 10% to determine what amount of drug may be present unless the USP monograph states otherwise. In the case of the commercially available 10-mg capsules, the USP monograph indicates that they may contain anywhere between 92.5% and 107.5% of the labeled strength. Therefore, a 10-mg capsule may contain anywhere from 9.25 to 10.75 mg of drug [6]. This same margin of error would be present when utilizing a compounded medication as well. Therefore, it does not make sense to compound any strength between 9 and 11 mg because the commercial capsule can be utilized to provide this dose. However, a 9-mg compounded capsule may contain anywhere from 8.1 to 9.9 mg. This may make it appropriate to compound. For a visual representation of this, see Figure 2.1. While these small milligram adjustments are clinically important with a narrow therapeutic index drug, they are less important in a medication like an antibiotic that has a large dosage range. In that case, a more substantial difference in strength is required to obtain a clinical benefit. From a broad application perspective, when considering the above example, we can assume that for a compounded strength to be significantly different from the commercial strength, there needs to be at least a 10% difference between the strength of the compound and the strength of the commercial product.

Eliminating Ingredients

Sometimes there is an FDA-approved product available in the desired strength and dosage form, but it contains an inactive ingredient that is toxic to the species, or a particular patient is not able to tolerate. In these cases, we are compounding to create a formulation that does not contain the problematic ingredient. The compound may or may not be the same dosage form and strength as the approved product.

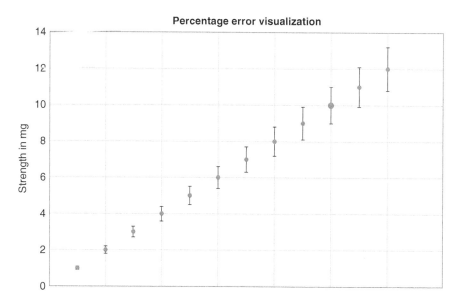

Figure 2.1 Graph showing ±10% error allowed for compounds. Strengths where error bars overlap will not produce a clinically significant difference.

Compounding to eliminate ingredients is often done to avoid xylitol that is present in commercial products. Xylitol is a sweetening agent that is not harmful to humans or other mammals except for dogs. In dogs, it can result in clinically significant hypoglycemia at doses as low as 50 mg/kg and acute liver failure at 500 mg/kg [7, 8]. Identifying the presence of xylitol can be difficult due to the variety of names it may be listed as such as birch sugar, wood sugar, and birch bark extract. The American Society for the Prevention of Cruelty to Animals recommends watching for any ingredients with "xyl" in the name as these are likely other names for xylitol. However, xylitol also might be listed under proprietary ingredients or included in "other sugar alcohols" [9]. Xylitol can be present in a variety of FDA-approved products, including toothpaste, mouthwash, chewing gum, sugar-free foods, candy, and lozenges. While it can also be found in a variety of human medication formulations, it is often found in oral liquids, orally disintegrating tablets, sublingual tablets, and chewable tablets. A common problematic product for veterinary patients is the commercially available gabapentin solutions which almost all contain xylitol making them toxic to canine patients. Therefore, compounded gabapentin suspensions are often used to ensure that patients do not receive a product containing xylitol. Another example of this benefit in practice is for a patient that has an allergy or intolerance to an excipient such as a dye. If the commercial product contains coloring, it may elicit an allergic response in the patient. Therefore, a product could be compounded to avoid the use of dyes.

Availability Issues

Even when a commercial product is acceptable from a dosage form, flavor, ingredient, and strength standpoint, backorders may still make compounding necessary. When an approved product is not available for purchase, a duplicate product can be compounded to meet medical needs that cannot be met utilizing another approved product. It is important to note that when the approved product becomes available again, the compounding of the duplicate must cease. Backordered products can be identified by reviewing the American Society of Health-System Pharmacists (ASHP) Drug Shortages List, and Current and Resolved Animal Drug Product lists available on the FDA website.

Appropriate Use of Compounded Medications

As discussed in the previous chapter, the use of compounded medications was legalized by the Animal Medicinal Drug Use Clarification Act (AMDUCA). The AMDUCA indicated that compounded medications should only be used when manufactured products were not appropriate. For a full decision tree on when compounding is legally appropriate in nonfood animal patients, refer to Figure 2.2 [10]. The American Veterinary Medical Association also has a stepwise decision algorithm on their website that can be used [11].

The AMDUCA emphasizes the need to use an FDA-approved product, if possible, for a couple of reasons. First, the approved product has higher reliability due to the restrictions of Current Good Manufacturing Practices (cGMPs). Additionally, as part of the approval process, the FDA has verified that the product is safe and effective when used as labeled and that sufficient information is provided with the product in the form of labeling and a package insert. The approval process also includes a review of the manufacturing process and facilities to ensure that the product can be reliably produced. To help emphasize the significance of these two points, what cGMP and FDA-approval requirements entail will be further elaborated on later in this chapter.

In addition to the safety, efficacy, and quality concerns, there is also concern about the potential for compounded medications to discourage pharmaceutical companies from introducing

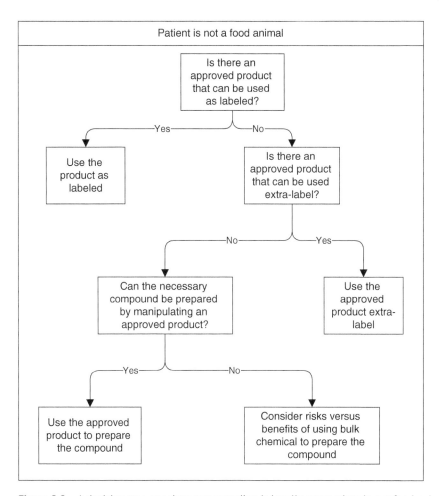

Figure 2.2 A decision tree on when compounding is legally appropriate in nonfood animal patients.

FDA-approved new animal drugs to the market or continuing to manufacture current products. This decreases the availability of approved products and proportionally increases the need for compounded medications. As mentioned above, compounded medications are less reliable than approved products. Although the FDA is aware that often commercial products do not meet the needs of specific patients, they are concerned that utilizing compounded products when a commercial product would be appropriate will disincentivize drug companies from pursuing approval of new animal drugs. The FDA-approval process and why it could potentially be thwarted by compounding will be further explained later in this chapter.

FDA-Approved Drugs

Throughout this text, there is a common theme that using an FDA-approved product should be first line and only after those options have been exhausted should a compounded medication be considered. To understand why FDA-approved drugs are considered first line, it is important to understand what goes into FDA approval.

The Food, Drug, and Cosmetic Act gives the FDA legal authority to approve drugs that are intended for use in either humans or animals. The legal definition of drugs is as follows:

> Articles recognized in the official United States Pharmacopoeia, official Homeopathic Pharmacopoeia of the United States, or official National Formulary, or any supplement to any of them; and articles intended for use in the diagnosis, cure, mitigation, treatment, or prevention of disease in man or other animals; and articles (other than food) intended to affect the structure or any function of the body of man or other animals . . . [12].

Basically, if something makes a claim to diagnose, treat, cure, mitigate, or prevent disease, then it is considered a drug. The Center for Veterinary Medicine (CVM) is the division of the FDA responsible for the approval of drugs intended for use in animals.

When a drug goes through the New Animal Drug Application (NADA) process, the drug sponsor must provide data to prove that the drug is safe and effective when used according to the label. Safe includes both the safety to the animal receiving the medication as well as the safety of any food products that may be made from the treated animal when the product is used in accordance with the labeling proposed in the application. Efficacy is based on its use for the indication that the NADA is submitted for. Extra-label indications and dosages of approved products have not been evaluated by the FDA for safety and efficacy [13].

During the approval process, the CVM also ensures that the drug's quality, strength, and purity are consistent from batch to batch, and evaluates the labeling, effect on the environment, and safety of the people who will be handling and administering the medication. There are five major technical sections of drug approval that encompass these points. They are as follows [13].

1) Target Animal Safety is evaluated through studies done in a small group of healthy animals of the target species. These studies look for potential side effects of the medication as well as the margin of safety when dosed higher and longer than intended.
2) Effectiveness is evaluated in a group of target animals that have the condition that the medication is designed to treat. These studies look to see if the medication effectively does what it is intended to do.
3) Human Food Safety is only evaluated for medications that are intended to be used in food-producing animals. For these medications, sponsors conduct studies to determine appropriate withdrawal times among other safety considerations.
4) Chemistry, Manufacturing, and Controls are evaluated by the sponsor as part of providing their plan for making the drug. The plan needs to include information about what ingredients will be used to make the drug, the source of the ingredients, the location where the drug will be manufactured, the packaging that will be used for the drug, storage conditions, and proposed expiration dating. This section also involves looking at the testing that will be done on final batches of the drug to ensure that it is consistently safe and high quality and determining when an inspection of the manufacturing facility is needed.
5) Environmental Impact is determined based on an Environmental Assessment that describes the amount of drug that is expected to be introduced into the environment and the potential effects. Generally, drugs for companion animals are less likely to present a significant environmental concern because they are being given to single patients and not entire herds or flocks.

The minor technical section of the NADA includes all other information such as published scientific literature, foreign experience for drugs approved outside of the United States, and studies that were not yet complete when the previous sections were submitted. Labeling is also included as a minor technical section. This includes the labeling on the immediate container, the outer packaging such as a carton, the package inserts, client information sheets, and the shipping label. All of this information is reviewed by the CVM for completeness and accuracy [13].

Finally, a Freedom of Information (FOI) Summary is published. This is a public document that summarizes the safety and efficacy data the CVM's approval was based on. The FOI summaries are readily available for the general public to view [13].

Generic drugs go through a similar approval process that involves an Abbreviated New Animal Drug Application (ANADA). In this process, there is no requirement to conduct new safety and efficacy studies because those were done with the original brand name product. To obtain CVM approval, generic drugs must be shown to have the same quality, effects, and intended uses as the approved brand name medication. As part of proving this information, the ANADA requires proof that the generic copy is bioequivalent to the brand. This means that the drug is absorbed and works the same way in the target species. The generic must also be proven identical to the brand name product with regard to active ingredient(s), strength, dosage form, and dosage regimen that includes the route of administration. Labeling must also be the same with the exception of items specific to the generic such as trade name, logo, and company name. The conclusion is that with these requirements, the generic will function in the same way as the brand, and they can be used interchangeably. This assumption can technically only be applied to the drug when used as labeled but is often extrapolated to extra-label uses in other species. It is also worth noting that human generic equivalents will only have bioavailability data to prove that absorption is the same as the brand name product in humans. This may or may not result in comparable absorption between the brand and generic products in veterinary patients [13].

Generic drugs are required to follow the same strict manufacturing processes that brand name products do. Testing is also required to ensure that there is batch-to-batch consistency regarding the safety and quality of the final product. Manufacturing sites for generic products are also required to undergo FDA inspection to ensure that they comply with cGMP standards.

Based on this strict approval process, the end user can be confident that all approved medications, regardless of whether they are brand name or generic products, will be safe and effective when used according to the labeling. However, this confidence does not come without a steep price tag. A study in 2015 found that it took an average of 6.5 years and $22.5 million to bring a companion animal drug to market with a new active ingredient. For drugs intended for food animals, the average time is 8.5 years and $30.5 million due to the increased safety studies needed to determine appropriate withdrawal times and safety of the human food supply. However, costs were found to be as high as $62 million [14]. Therefore, which drugs to bring to market is a strategic decision for companies, and not everything needed for treating veterinary patients will be developed as an approved drug. The result is that we rely on compounding to fill the gaps where manufactured products fail.

Compounded Medication Risks

Compounded medications are not FDA-approved products; therefore, they do not come with the peace of mind inherent to products that have gone through the rigorous FDA-approval process. While there may be studies for some compounded medications, there is no requirement to prove safety and efficacy for compounded products. Whether or not the requirements regarding manufacturing processes are required to be followed for compounded medications depends on whether that compound is being made in a 503a pharmacy or 503b facility. With regards to the associated

Table 2.2 USP and cGMP requirements for final testing and beyond-use/expiration dates.

	USP [15] requirements (503a)[a]	cGMP [16] requirements (503b)
Release testing	Sterility and endotoxin testing may be required based on beyond-use date. No other testing required.	Each batch requires testing to verify it contains the correct active ingredient and quantity and is sterile if it's a dosage form that requires sterility.
Beyond-use date/ expiration date determination	Can use USP default dating, but stability testing required (or referencing a study done elsewhere) if extended beyond the default dating.	Must be determined based on stability testing as defined in cGMP regulations.

[a] State laws may vary on these requirements.

risks, release testing and beyond use date (BUD) determination have a significant impact. Table 2.2 provides a basic comparison of the USP versus cGMP requirements for release testing and BUD determination. Chapter 1 talks about the applicability of 503b facilities in veterinary medicine and for nonsterile compounds. This chapter will discuss what it means for a compound to come from a 503b facility.

Compounded (USP) Versus Manufactured (cGMP)

cGMPs are codified in the Code of Federal Regulations Title 21 Parts 210 and 211. Part 211 consists of the following 11 subparts.

– Subpart A – General Provisions
– Subpart B – Organization and Personnel
– Subpart C – Buildings and Facilities
– Subpart D – Equipment
– Subpart E – Control of Components and Drug Product Containers and Closures
– Subpart F – Production and Process Controls
– Subpart G – Packaging and Labeling Control
– Subpart H – Holding and Distribution
– Subpart I – Laboratory Controls
– Subpart J – Records and Reports
– Subpart K – Returned and Salvaged Drug Products

These sections of the Code of Federal Regulations detail the required processes and procedures and documentation in each of these areas. As these are the same requirements put in place for manufactured products, they are designed to be done on a large scale. It would not be practical or feasible to employ these requirements on an individual patient scale. One requirement included in cGMP is that all the components must be tested to verify identity, and that they conform with written specifications for purity, strength, and quality. Containers and closures also need to be tested to ensure that they conform with written specifications. One example of the requirements for procedures can be found in Subpart F. It states that procedures detailing production and process control must be in place and approved by a quality control unit. Once approved, all the deviations from the stated procedures must be documented and justified. These procedures must include built in double checks. For example, when components are added to a batch, it must be done by one person and verified by another to ensure that there are two sets of eyes. If components are added using automated equipment, then a single human verification step is required [16].

USP standards are split into chapters based on whether the compounded product is a sterile or nonsterile preparation with additional requirements for hazardous drugs. The purpose of these USP standards is to provide good compounding practices for preparing sterile (USP <797>) and nonsterile (USP <795>) preparations. By design, USP standards are written to provide a framework for producing high-quality compounded medications on a patient-specific scale. They were not designed for large-scale production like cGMP standards are, which allows for more flexibility to make small batches of meds tailored to the needs of a specific patient. However, that increased flexibility comes with trade-offs regarding risks.

Compounds prepared under USP standards (503a facilities or traditional pharmacies) have the following inherent risks.

- Incorrect potency: The compound contains either more or less active ingredient than stated on the label. The compounding process has several points where ingredient loss can occur to the point that the correct amount is weighed/measured, yet the final product does not contain enough active ingredient. On the converse, a decimal point could be transposed, or a scale read incorrectly leading to too much or too little active ingredient. There could also be incorrect amounts of inactive ingredients. While likely less obvious, ingredient amounts of excipients can negatively impact the concentration, stability, or absorption of a compounded product.
- Incorrect ingredient: The wrong medication was put into the compound. Many compounding ingredients are white powders, and depending on the verification process, an ingredient mix up that leads to an incorrect ingredient or switching the strengths of two active ingredients could occur. Incorrect excipients could also be introduced leading to stability and/or absorption problems.
- Lack of stability: The active ingredient degrades before the beyond-use date (BUD) is reached. USP provides default BUDs that are generally short enough that drug degradation and microbial contamination will not occur during the use period of the product. However, that is not guaranteed. There is also concern about whether extended dates are based on true stability-indicating assays or if they are based on potency over time. The latter is not sufficient for determining extended BUDs. This concept will be covered in more detail in Chapter 3.
- Lack of efficacy: The compound is prepared correctly, but it does not produce the intended effect in the patient. This may be because the bioavailability (amount absorbed) is too low, the product was prepared incorrectly, or the product degraded too quickly.
- Lack of safety: The compound is prepared correctly, but there is something that makes it unsafe for the patient. This could be an inactive ingredient, dose, or route that has a high potential of causing harm to a patient.
- Excessive microbial growth or lack of sterility: Nonsterile compounds are exactly as the name implies, not sterile. However, they still need to have adequate preservatives or short enough dating that excessive microbial growth does not occur while the medication is in use. Sterile products, on the other hand, need to be sterile. While a sterile environment that complies with USP <797> greatly increases the probability that the final product will be sterile, there is still the potential for contamination to occur resulting in a final product that is not actually sterile. Even if batch testing is done and a certain percentage of the batch is determined to be sterile, there is still the potential (although less than without any testing) that there is contamination in an item that was not tested as contamination is not uniformly distributed.

Compounded medications prepared under cGMP (503b or outsourcing facilities) are not FDA approved, which means they still have some inherent risks. However, the additional safeguards put in place in the manufacturing process address some of the concerns that are present when compounds are prepared based on USP standards. The FDA-approval process is where safety and efficacy are proven before the drug can be marketed. Since these are not FDA-approved products, there is no requirement to prove safety and efficacy. However, independent researchers or 503b companies may decide to study and publish these data which would decrease the concern. The final testing that is required by cGMP requires testing a percentage of each batch prior to release. This testing verifies the correct identity and potency of the active ingredient as well as sterility if the product is marketed as sterile. There are also requirements that the 503b facility has proven that the preparation process yields a consistently uniform batch as well as that the formulation has sufficient stability for the expiration date given. For sterility, there is potential that the tested products are sterile, but other products in the batch are contaminated. However, the large-scale manufacturing process designed to ensure consistency and repeatability between batches decreases that risk. Owing to these cGMP requirements, efficacy and safety data obtained from studies of 503b products have the potential to be more universally applicable than safety and efficacy studies on 503a compounded products, which may have significant batch-to-batch variability.

Risks Associated with Compounded Medications – A Look at the Literature

There is no question that compounded medications provide essential treatment for patients that would not be effectively treated without them. It is also clear based on the above sections that the theoretical risks of compounded medications are potentially severe. However, it can be easy to give a nod to the news stories discussed in Chapter 1 and assume that it is highly unlikely anything like that would happen to one of your patients. Is that reality or is the likelihood of something going wrong with a compound much higher than the infrequent news stories may lead us to believe? This section will summarize the findings from several studies and surveys attempting to answer this question from both the human and veterinary perspectives. It is important to keep in mind that a quality compounding pharmacy will have a process where formulations prepared are developed in conjunction with a literature review to ensure that potential problems, such as lack of efficacy, are identified. However, there are frequently compounding pharmacies that will prepare something because a veterinarian requests it and fail to do their own literature review assuming that the veterinarian has reviewed the available information and believes it will be effective.

Studies Showing Incorrect Potency

A study by Umstead et al. [17] evaluated compounded cyclosporine A capsules and solution. The study looked at two different strengths of capsules (10 and 300 mg) and solutions (50 and 150 mg/ml) from five pharmacies as well as using five positive controls (Atopica 10-mg and 100-mg capsules and human generic 50-mg and 100-mg capsules and 100-mg/ml solution). The pharmacies included two nationally known compounding pharmacies, two less well-known online compounding pharmacies, and a local compounding pharmacy. The compounded medications were ordered for clinic stock and were ordered three separate times.

Notable results included the following.

- The study found that the accuracy of these positive controls ranged from 92% to 103%, which is to be expected based on requirements for manufactured products.
- Most of the compounded liquids that were indicated to be solutions were actually suspensions based on the visible particles present.
- No pharmacy objected to the requested 10-mg capsules being the same strength as a commercially available product.
- For the 50-mg/ml liquid compound, the samples from all the pharmacies failed to fall within the allowed ±10%, and for the 150 mg/ml, the samples from two pharmacies failed to fall within ±10%.
- For the 10-mg capsules, the samples from one pharmacy failed to fall within the allowed ±10%. All of the 300-mg capsule samples were within ±10% of the labeled strength.

A case report by Thompson et al. [18] explores the effects of clenbuterol toxicosis on three Quarter Horse racehorses. This toxicosis occurred 12–24 hours after the oral administration of a compounded clenbuterol solution that was labeled to contain 72.5 mcg/ml of clenbuterol. The horses had previously been receiving the FDA-approved 72.5-mcg/ml clenbuterol syrup without issue, and this was the first administration of the compounded product. It is suspected that several other horses received this same product and had similar negative reactions. Of the three horses discussed in the case report, two were euthanized due to laminitis, acute renal failure, cardiomyopathy, and rhabdomyolysis. Based on product analysis, the compounded product was found to contain 5 mg/ml of clenbuterol, which is about 70 times more concentrated than the approved product and the labeled strength of the compounded product administered.

A case report by McConkey et al. [19] discusses two canine patients receiving compounded antiepileptic medications. In the second case in this report, a dog experienced bromide toxicity after a compounding error resulted in a potassium bromide product containing five times the stated amount of bromide.

Since the accurate dosing of chemotherapy medications is essential for safe and effective treatment, compounded products are frequently utilized to obtain the desired dosage. However, that logic relies on the assumption that the compounded product is accurately formulated and remains stable throughout its shelf life. To that end, several studies have looked at the potency and stability of compounded chemotherapy agents.

A 2016 study by Robat and Budde [20] evaluated the potency of compounded cyclophosphamide capsules. Compounded capsules were obtained from five separate pharmacies at two separate time points. Four of these pharmacies were large, national compounding pharmacies and one was a local pharmacy. Of the national pharmacies, two specialized in veterinary compounding. Four out of 10 samples (40%) failed to fall within ±10% of the labeled strength with potency ranging from 68.3% to 106% of the labeled strength. This study also noted wide variability in cost with no correlation between cost and potency results.

A 2017 study by Burton et al. [21] looked at the potency of compounded chlorambucil, melphalan, and cyclophosphamide. Six pharmacies were chosen based on advertisements in national veterinary publications. This study found chlorambucil potency ranged from 71% to 104%, melphalan potency ranged from 58% to 109%, and cyclophosphamide potency ranged from 92% to 107% of the labeled strength. Another study from this group [22] looked at the frequency of neutropenia in patients receiving an FDA-approved lomustine formulation compared to those patients receiving a compounded formulation. The study found that all the dogs that received the FDA-approved product were neutropenic following treatment, while only 25% of the dogs receiving the compounded product became neutropenic. This finding led the group to evaluate the potency of lomustine from five compounding pharmacies. They found potency ranged from 50% to 115% with only one of the five products being within ±10% of the labeled strength.

KuKanich et al. [23] also looked at the potency of compounded lomustine capsules. This study evaluated two capsule formulations from three compounding pharmacies compared to the manufactured product. The compounded capsule potency ranged from 59% to 95% of the labeled strength and was outside of the allowed ±10% in 7/10 samples. In contrast, the FDA-approved product potency ranged from 104% to 110% of the labeled strength.

Famciclovir is a commonly compounded medication that has been evaluated in multiple studies. Johnson et al. [24] evaluated the potency of various compounded formulations including multiple concentrations of oral oil suspension, oral paste, and tablets. Compounds were obtained from a single national veterinary compounding pharmacy. This study found that when the products arrived from the compounding pharmacy, 5 out of 12 oral suspensions, and 3 out of 3 oral pastes were outside of ±10% of the labeled strength. The tablets were within the acceptable range.

O'Leary et al. [25] also looked at compounded famciclovir. Their study evaluated accuracy, precision, and consistency in the drug content of oral liquid formulations. A total of 30 preparations split between two strengths (250 and 400 mg/ml) were analyzed and compared to the FDA-approved tablets. The samples were analyzed at time 0 and then again on days 14 and 28. When looking at all the time points, 15 of the 63 250-mg/ml samples analyzed were within ±10% of the labeled strength and none of the 27 400-mg/ml samples fell within ±10%.

Doxycycline is another commonly studied compounded medication. KuKanich et al. [26] looked at compounded doxycycline hyclate tablets, chews, and doxycycline calcium oral liquids compared to FDA-approved products. Formulations were evaluated on days 1 and 21. On day 1, 9 (60%) of the 15 compounded tablets were within the acceptable range; 5 (33%) of the 15 chews were within the acceptable range, and none of the three liquid preparations were within the acceptable range. On day 21, none of the compounded products met USP standards.

A study by Laporte et al. [27] evaluated the quality of compounded fluconazole products. Capsules and oral suspensions were obtained from four veterinary compounding pharmacies located in the United States. The products were ordered three separate times form each of the pharmacies. The study found that seven of the eight capsules evaluated had acceptable accuracy (±10% of labeled strength). However, only one of the eight suspensions evaluated was found to have acceptable accuracy.

A 2012 study by Scott-Moncrieff et al. [28] evaluated commercially manufactured PZI insulin versus compounded PZI insulin from multiple pharmacies. In this study, 16 vials of commercially manufactured PZI insulin and 8 vials each from 12 compounding pharmacies were evaluated. Out of the 96 vials of compounded PZI tested, only 13 (13.5%) met the USP specifications for PZI insulin, whereas all the manufactured vials met the specifications. The USP specifications evaluated in this study included appearance, endotoxin concentration, crystal size, insulin concentration in the supernatant, pH, zinc content, total insulin concentration, and the species of insulin origin.

A study by Stanley et al. [29] looked at compounded versus FDA-approved formulations of ketoprofen, amikacin, and boldenone. For the ketoprofen, one compound out of the 10 evaluated was only about 50% of the labeled strength. For the compounded amikacin, the potency was widely variable with a range of 59–140% of the labeled strength with none being within ±10% of the labeled strength. For the boldenone, two compounded products were outside of the 10% range, but both were within 15% of the labeled strength. However, one compounded boldenone had total impurity levels of about 5%, which is significantly higher than the approximately 1% found in the FDA-approved products. For trilostane, a study by Cook et al. [30] looked at the potency of compounded trilostane capsules. The study evaluated 96 batches of the compounded trilostane and found that 38% were outside of the acceptance criteria (90–105% of labeled strength) with a range of 39–152.6% of labeled strength.

Problems with the potency of compounded products are not limited to veterinary compounding. Shah et al. [31] evaluated the potency and content uniformity of topical 2% diltiazem hydrochloride compounded for anal fissure treatment in human patients. In this study, 36 prescriptions for diltiazem cream were filled by 12 pharmacies. Six of the pharmacies prepared an ointment instead of a cream. Out of the 36 prescriptions, five were suprapotent ranging from 117.2% to 128.5% of the labeled strength, and 13 were subpotent ranging from 34.8% to 89.8% of the labeled strength. Fourteen of the preparations lacked sufficient compound uniformity by USP definitions. Out of the 12 pharmacies included, 9 failed potency or content uniformity for at least 1 of the 3 prescriptions filled.

In a study done by Meyer et al. [32], six pharmacies and six student pharmacists prepared a compounded 25-mcg/ml levothyroxine oral liquid formulation on two separate occasions. These preparations were tested for potency. On day 3 after compounding, the formulations prepared by compounding pharmacies ranged from 77% to 93% of labeled strength, and those prepared by student pharmacists ranged from 98% to 113% of labeled strength.

Studies Showing Lack of Stability

In the other case reported by McConkey et al. [19], a dog received a compounded, flavored phenobarbital solution. In this case, the product deteriorated below the 90% acceptable limit prior to the stated beyond-use date. In this patient, increased seizure activity and corresponding low phenobarbital trough levels were noted despite increased dosages. This solution was stated to have a three-month beyond-use date, but when tested after only half of the stated shelf life, the product was found to have 2.5 mg/ml of phenobarbital despite the label stating a concentration of 5 mg/ml.

The 2016 Robat and Budde [20] study also evaluated the stability of compounded cyclophosphamide capsules at 60 days post receipt. Compounded capsules were obtained from five separate pharmacies, four of which were large, national compounding pharmacies and one was a local pharmacy. Two of the national pharmacies specialized in veterinary compounding. This study found that four of the five samples had adequate stability at 60 days.

Papich et al. [33] looked at doxycycline concentration over time. This study evaluated doxycycline liquid formulations prepared from doxycycline hyclate tablets. The liquid compounds stayed within ±10% of the labeled strength for the first seven days of the study. However, by day 14, the doxycycline concentrations had significantly decreased to less than 20% of the labeled strength.

Stability problems are also not limited to veterinary compounding. In a study of levothyroxine suspension by Boulton et al. [34], they found that there was significant drug degradation after eight days of refrigerated storage regardless of whether the suspension was made with or without preservative.

Studies Showing Lack of Efficacy

Depending on the drug in question, product efficacy can be more difficult to determine. However, testing such as plasma levels of drug and dissolution characteristics have been used for a couple medications to determine efficacy compared to FDA-approved versions of the medication. One of these drugs is itraconazole that has been evaluated in several studies with similar results. A study by Molter et al. [35] found that after two months of treatment with compounded itraconazole in a parrot, disease progression was noted and plasma itraconazole levels were undetectable. A sample of the compounded product was analyzed and found to contain the labeled concentration of 50 mg/ml. Therefore, the study concluded that the compounded product was not effectively absorbed. Smith et al. [36] evaluated itraconazole pharmacokinetics in penguins using a two-way crossover design. The study measured plasma itraconazole concentrations at time 0 and then 20 minutes, 40 minutes, and 1, 2, 4, 6, 8, and 12 hours after drug administration. The study noted significant differences in absorption between the commercial and compounded products with the compounded product significantly lower. The compounded product was also noted to have more variable and inconsistent absorption. Mawby et al. evaluated the absorption of compounded itraconazole in cats [37] and dogs [38]. In both studies, it was noted that the compounded products showed poor and inconsistent absorption compared to the FDA-approved products. These findings are similar to those found in the penguin study noted above. The results of these studies indicate that compounded itraconazole products are ineffective in a variety of species.

For trilostane, a study by Cook et al. [30] looked at the dissolution characteristics of compounded trilostane capsules. For dissolution, 20% of the compounded products did not meet the acceptance criteria of greater than or equal to 70% dissolution at 75 minutes. Of the five pharmacies from which compounded product was obtained, three of them met the dissolution criteria for all batches, but two failed to meet the criteria for at least 50% of the batches tested. The authors concluded that this indicates that there may be decreased efficacy of the compounded product compared to the FDA-approved product. A lower dissolution rate potentially has clinical significance because it refers to the rate that a solution is formed, and drug must be dissolved before it can be absorbed.

Another medication where efficacy of the compounded product compared to the FDA-approved product frequently comes into question is omeprazole paste for use in horses. A study by Merritt et al. [39] evaluated the gastric acid inhibition of FDA-approved GastroGard compared to compounded omeprazole from three pharmacies. This study found that only the FDA-approved product and one other preparation had a significant change in the variables of question. Another omeprazole study by Nieto et al. [40] evaluated a compounded omeprazole suspension compared to the FDA-approved product. They found the compounded product to be ineffective of healing ulcers in actively training racehorses, whereas the FDA-approved product was effective in this population.

Risks Associated with Specific Types of Compounds

While risks such as incorrect drug concentration or lack of stability are inherent with all the compounded medications, some compounded formulations include additional risks specific to the drug or dosage form. Dosage forms that are being administered to a sterile site, such as ophthalmic and injectable products, have the additional risk that they may not be sterile. One study found the contamination rate to be 5.2% with technician-prepared preparations having a slightly higher contamination rate compared with pharmacist-prepared preparations (6.2% versus 4.4%) [41]. Another study found that the environment in which sterile compounds are prepared impacted the contamination rate. In a study by Stucki et al. [42], 1500 sterile syringe preparations were prepared in three separate environments. None of the syringes prepared in a cleanroom were contaminated, while 6% prepared in an operating room and 16% prepared in a ward space were contaminated. Even if the finished sterile preparations have testing done on a percentage of the batch, contamination may not be spread evenly throughout the batch still creating the potential that there may be contaminated units in a larger batch that passed sterility testing. When batches are released of either manufactured or compounded sterile products and later determined to have contamination, a recall is issued. Drug recalls can be viewed on the FDA site at https://www.fda.gov/drugs/drug-safety-and-availability/drug-recalls. USP <797> is designed to outline best practices to prevent contamination of sterile preparations while still being feasible on a patient-specific scale. This chapter includes information on facility design for sterile compounding, appropriate personal protective equipment, and quality control. While these may appear stringent, the need to make them feasible on a small scale means that there are still opportunities for contamination and the associated negative effects to occur.

Another risk that warrants consideration is the risk associated with hazardous drugs, both from the standpoint of the person preparing the compound as well as the person administering it. Many nonsterile hazardous drugs are formulated in such a way that there is some level of protection built in. This is often by formulating the drug into a capsule or applying a protective coating to the outside of tablets. Both formulations serve to contain the hazardous drug and, therefore, limit the exposure of those administering it. However, when we start to manipulate these hazardous drugs and create new dosage forms, human exposure to hazardous drugs is increased. For example, if a chemotherapy agent is formulated into an oral liquid, there was the potential for chemotherapy exposure for the person(s) preparing the liquid. There is also an increased likelihood of the client being exposed to chemotherapy through the normal use of this compound. From the standpoint of protecting the person doing the compounding, USP has provided minimum best practices in General Chapter <800>, which includes information such as compounding facility requirements. The National Institute for Occupational Safety and Health has provided criteria for identifying hazardous drugs. However, USP does not address the protection of those handling the medication once it leaves the compounding/healthcare facility. Therefore, it is a joint responsibility of the person preparing the compound as well as the veterinarian prescribing it to ensure that the client understands the potential hazards and how dosage form may potentially contribute. In general, capsules represent the lowest risk of exposure followed by tablets and then pastes and liquids. It is important to note that opening capsules or splitting/crushing tablets will significantly increase the risk of exposure potentially to a higher level than liquids. The full requirements of hazardous drug handling are outside the scope of this book. However, simply because the medication is contained in packaging such as a vial or a blister pack does not mean that the person handling it is free from exposure. In 2018, the ASHP published guidelines on handling hazardous drugs. These guidelines [43] include summaries of multiple studies showing a risk of exposure in job classifications besides those preparing or administering chemotherapy medications. The studies included in the ASHP guidelines emphasize the following points.

- Hazardous drug contamination is widespread throughout preparation and administration areas, and this has not improved much between studies conducted in 1999 and in 2010 despite the increased use of Class II biological safety cabinets.
- Healthcare workers in drug administration settings may have detectable chemotherapy levels in their urine despite not being involved in chemotherapy administration. Detectable chemotherapy levels can also be identified in workers in areas where there is no chemotherapy preparation or administration such as shipping/receiving.
- Training on safe hazardous drug handling decreased the risk of chemotherapy absorption.
- Dermal contact with contaminated surfaces is the primary route of exposure in workers not involved in preparation or administration.
- When chemotherapy drugs are received in a pharmacy contamination has been found on the outside of vials, inside of packing cartons, package inserts, and the outside of tablet blister packs.

Active Ingredient Source Decisions

Another compounding decision that can introduce risk is whether to prepare the compound using bulk chemical (aka active pharmaceutical ingredient or API) versus the approved product as the source of the active ingredient(s). Chapter 1 discusses how AMDUCA defines compounded drugs as being prepared by modifying approved products. While there is risk associated with the use of bulk chemicals as the active ingredient source, there are also risks to using the commercial product as the active ingredient source. Therefore, active ingredient source requires a risk–benefit analysis. Table 2.3 outlines the risks and benefits associated with bulk chemicals versus commercial products when used as the active ingredient source.

When considering the quality of your active ingredients, there are different things to look at depending on if it is an approved product or a bulk chemical. For approved products, you can be assured that cGMP requirements were followed in its production, and therefore, the final product has been tested and shown to meet the USP monograph requirements for that medication. USP monographs provide the quality expectations for a drug and the tests to verify that the drugs meet those requirements. Typically, these requirements include that the amount of active drug must be within ±10% of the labeled strength with a few drugs having wider or narrower allowed margins of error.

For bulk chemicals, they should be manufactured in FDA-approved facilities, but the end-product testing is different since the product is not a finished medication. Therefore, these products should come with a certificate of analysis (CoA) that lists all of the USP monograph requirements for that active ingredient and how the prepared drug compares. CoAs are lot specific since each lot must be tested for USP compliance. All the bulk chemical active ingredients must

Table 2.3 Benefits and risks of using approved products versus bulk chemicals as the active ingredient source for compounding.

Approved products		Bulk chemicals	
Benefits	**Risks**	**Benefits**	**Risks**
– Prepared under cGMP guidelines which requires evaluating potency and stability – Legally accepted through AMDUCA – Distinctive appearance and packaging decreases risk of selecting incorrect drug	– Unknown potency within allowed margin of error – Inactive ingredients can cause formulation problems – Patient may have an allergy or intolerance to inactive ingredient – Difficult to increase concentration of a commercial product – Required manipulations of commercial products (e.g. opening capsules) may increase the risk of hazardous drug exposure by compounding personnel	– High-quality powders are prepared under cGMP guidelines – Certificate of analysis shows exact amounts of drug and impurities – No additional excipients to affect final formulation	– Wide range of quality means benefits may not always be true – Powders and packaging often look very similar to each other which increases the risk of error

have the CoA provided or have a place online for the product recipient to download the CoA for the lot of product received. The CoA should be reviewed for each received bulk chemical active ingredient. However, there is not a requirement for 503a pharmacies to independently test the chemical to verify the accuracy of the CoA.

Patient-Specific Compounding Versus Office Use Compounding

How many patients a specific lot of compounded medication will be distributed to also plays a role in determining the potential risk. The potential risks that are present are the same whether the compound is made for one patient or shipped throughout the country as office stock. However, the negative effects if the risk occurs become more significant as more patients receive the defective product. This is because we assume that when something like incorrect drug concentration occurs, it is human error at a single point in time, so if the same compound is made in the future, the potential that the same error occurred again is no more or less likely than any other time. Consider the following example that illustrates why office use is considered higher risk than patient-specific compounding.

> A compounding pharmacy prepares a large batch of a compounded steroid injection for epidural administration. Vials from this batch are distributed to healthcare facilities across the country for administration to future patients as needed (i.e. office stock use). However, in this case, there was fungal growth occurring in the ventilation system of the cleanroom used to prepare the batch resulting in fungal contamination in many vials. This resulted in significant morbidity and mortality across the country.
>
> When we consider this case, the compound was something legitimate to compound and it is something facilities needed to have on hand versus ordering per patient. Therefore, the office use was potentially appropriate. There is no reason to believe that if a small batch of this medication was prepared for one or two patients needing it, they would have fared any better as the lack of sterility does not appear to be related to batch size. However, the morbidity and mortality would have been much smaller scale than this case, which is a basic summary of what happened with the fungal meningitis outbreak discussed in Chapter 1.

The above case example illustrates why office use compounding is subject to more restrictions and oversight than patient-specific compounding. Despite the risks, there are still reasons why office stock is necessary in veterinary medicine. For medications like metronidazole that may need to be compounded for puppies, it is desirable to start the medication the day the need is determined versus waiting several days for a compounded medication to be shipped. Another instance is for sterile compounds designed to be administered in-house during surgical procedures. These are medications that need to be kept on hand to use for surgeries, which may not always be scheduled.

In some cases, the need for office stock and the associated risks could be balanced by considering in-house compounding. For the metronidazole example above, this could potentially be compounded by the veterinarian when needed. This would remove the delay of not having it as office stock but allow it to be prepared in a patient-specific manner. However, that option introduces the risks associated with in-house compounding. These concerns fall into the same risk groups discussed earlier in this chapter. However, some risks have the potential to be more likely when compounded medications are not prepared in a pharmacy setting. Therefore, it is important to acknowledge these and develop a plan to reduce the risk. While risks such as safety and efficacy concerns are likely in any setting, the following risks are those that will require additional risk mitigation strategies when compounding in-house versus using a high-quality compounding pharmacy.

- Incorrect potency: As discussed earlier in the chapter, the compounding process has several points where ingredient loss can occur to the point that the correct amount is weighed/measured, yet the final product does not contain enough active ingredient. Compounding pharmacists are trained to address these ingredient loss concerns through appropriate technique. Since veterinarians receive less training on medication compounding, this is an area that warrants awareness and attention. Chapter 6 provides additional information on these techniques.
- Lack of sterility: Sterile products need to be sterile. While a sterile environment that complies with USP <797> greatly increases the probability that the final product will be sterile, there is still the potential for contamination to occur resulting in a final product that is not actually sterile. Owing to the high risk that contaminated sterile products pose, the authors recommend that sterile compounds not intended for immediate use only be prepared in facilities that are fully compliant with USP <797> standards.

Another gray area is the concept of anticipatory compounding. Anticipatory compounding occurs when a pharmacy makes a batch of a compounded medication in anticipation of getting prescriptions requiring that medication within the near future. In this case, the amount prepared in advance is based on historical dispensing history from that pharmacy. An example of this would be preparing a batch of compounded capsules utilizing a 300-count capsule machine. The pharmacy may only need 20 of these capsules that day, but based on previous dispensing trends, they anticipate that they will dispense all 300 capsules within the next few weeks. The difference between anticipatory compounding and office stock is that the compounded medication will not leave the pharmacy until there is a patient-specific prescription for it. Therefore, anticipatory compounding is generally lumped in with patient-specific compounding from a regulatory standpoint. From a risk standpoint, anticipatory compounding falls between patient-specific compounding and office use compounding. With anticipatory compounding, a large batch is made with the intent that it will be distributed to several patients, which is also the case with office stock meaning that the risk of a compounding error spreading to many patients is increased. However, since the compounded medication is only leaving the pharmacy for specific patients, the pharmacy is better able to contact all the clients using the defective compound when adverse effects are reported. This is due to the requirement that the lot number dispensed for a compounded medication be documented for each prescription. The pharmacy is then able to tie a specific lot number to a specific formulation record allowing tracking down to what lot of each ingredient was used. When compounds are sold for office use, this ability to quickly track every patient that received a compound when an error is discovered is less reliable. An example of this is that if an ingredient used in a compound is recalled, a pharmacy will be able to track everyone that has received a compound using the recalled lot of the ingredient. However, if some of the compounds made with that recalled ingredient were sold as office stock, the pharmacy would only be able to track the compounds as far as the veterinary clinic they were sold to. It would be up to the veterinarian to determine which patients received the compound containing the recalled ingredient.

Adverse Event Reporting

The reporting of adverse events that occur and are potentially linked to medications is important to ensure that underlying issues are discovered. This is true regardless of whether the medication is a compound or an approved product. For approved products, they go through phase 4 of drug approval, which is where the drug is marketed, and adverse effects are closely tracked. This provides the opportunity to identify adverse effects that may be so rare they were not appreciated in the pre-marketing studies that were conducted. For compounded products, we do not have anywhere near the number of safety studies that approved products do and different formulations of the same drug may result in a different set of potential adverse effects. Therefore, it is important that we monitor and track these adverse effects. It will likely require several people reporting issues for it to be tied to a specific drug, formulation, or source, so even if reporting may not seem significant for your specific issue, everyone's small adverse effects that are reported can add up to a significant finding.

Problems that should be reported include side effects in patients receiving the medication, side effects in people exposed to the drug through administration or preparation, defects such as broken product seals, lack of efficacy, and medication errors. It is important to note that only problems with products regulated by the FDA should be reported to the FDA. Veterinary biologics, which include vaccines, and many flea and tick products are not regulated by the FDA. Since these products are not typically compounded, how to report adverse events for non-FDA products will not be discussed in this text. The method for reporting adverse events for FDA-regulated products varies by product type [44].

- Drugs that are FDA-approved or indexed for animals: The preferred method is to contact the drug company and ask to speak to a technical services representative to report an adverse drug event. Drug companies are required to submit adverse drug event reports to the FDA. Alternatively, you can submit Form FDA 1932a directly to the FDA.
- Drugs not approved for animals (human-labeled products and compounds): Download and complete Form FDA 1932a and submit to the FDA as directed on the form. Additional details on completing this form can be found on the FDA webpage How to Report Animal Drug and Device Side Effects and Product Problems.

Adverse event report data are made available to the public on openFDA.gov, which includes data from January 1, 1987. The data set is updated quarterly. The data set includes reports of adverse events in animal patients associated with approved animal drugs, drugs not approved in animals (human-labeled drugs), compounded drugs, and devices. A challenge to accessing these data is that the platform is designed to be used by those familiar with application programming interfaces, so it is not intuitive for those unfamiliar with APIs. To that end, there are independent applications that have been designed to mine the data from openFDA [45]. Once these have been verified by the FDA to be legitimate, they are included on the openFDA Apps webpage. At the time of writing, the listed app available for mining veterinary adverse event data is AdverseVeterinaryEvents. com (AVE).

Identifying Potential Formulation Issues

Often formulation and stability problems are invisible when simply looking at the product. However, product appearance changes should never be ignored because sometimes problems can result in visible changes to the product. Any product having a significantly different appearance than before (i.e. new color) should warrant a call to the pharmacy to verify that the new appearance is intentional and does not indicate a potential problem. This change could be intentional on the part of the pharmacy, or it could indicate that the wrong strength or drug was provided. Many compounding pharmacies will color-code their tablet and capsule compounds to identify the active ingredient and/or the strength. For example, a pharmacy may decide that every time gabapentin 50-mg capsules are compounded, bright pink gelatin capsules will be used, and every time 25-mg gabapentin capsules are compounded, the gelatin capsules used will be bright pink on top and clear on the bottom. This is an example of the pharmacy color-coding gabapentin with bright pink and then color-coding the different strengths with one having a partially clear capsule. For pharmacies that do this, if you tell them what product you expected to get and the color of the one you received, they can quickly determine if the correct product was provided. However, this color-coding system can be imprecise as there is a finite number of gelatin capsule colors available, and they are subject to supply issues necessitating color substitutions. Alternatively, pharmacies could color the active drug powder prior to putting it into clear capsules as an indicator of the medication. This coloring process is similar to what would be done with tablet coloring.

Beyond the identity of the medication, a change in color can indicate a stability problem. This is most likely to occur in liquid formulations. Some medications are known to change color during their appropriate duration of use. For example, Convenia (cefovecin) starts off as a pale yellow and becomes a darker orange the closer it gets to the use by date after reconstitution. If color change is noted in a compound during the use duration, it is beneficial to contact the pharmacy or research if color change is expected for that medication. An example of color change problems is ceftazidime otic. Otic compounds at the time of writing default to a 30 day beyond-use date at room temperature per USP. This particular otic compound was noted to go from clear to yellow to orange color during the 30 days. Further research found that some color change to yellow is expected, but the orange color seen during the second half of the month indicated stability problems because ceftazidime degrades quickly at room temperature. Therefore, to keep this compound stable, it needs to be stored in the refrigerator. The color change prompted additional investigation in this case.

A change in smell can also indicate stability problems. If a compound is flavored, it should smell like the flavor. Regardless of whether flavor is added, the smell should remain the same throughout the duration of use. Another visual indicator is the integrity of the tablet or capsule. If a capsule is cracking or a tablet is crumbling, this is an indicator that there is a potential stability issue. When tablets crumble, it is often due to absorbing moisture from the air and causing the tablet to expand and crumble. When capsules crack, it can also be a sign of instability.

For liquids, note if the product is a suspension or solution initially. Solutions are completely clear, whereas suspensions will have visible drug distributed throughout. If a formerly clear solution starts having a precipitant that is a sign of a potential problem. For suspensions, the suspended drug is expected to settle to the bottom after a period of time. However, it should be evenly distributed by shaking. If the drug cakes at the bottom and is not redistributed after shaking, the suspension will no longer provide the expected concentration of drug.

Another important observation that can assist with identifying a potential problem is whether the expected response is achieved. In the lomustine study [22] and seizure case reports [19] described above, a lack of the intended response or unexpected adverse effects were the indicators that led the authors to look closer into the quality of the compounded medications.

Drugs Recalls

Recalls are a voluntary action that a manufacturer or distributor can take to meet their responsibility to protect the public health from products that present a risk of injury or are otherwise defective. The FDA can also request a product be recalled if the company has not requested a recall, and there is sufficient reason to believe a health risk exists. If the company refuses to complete the requested recall, then the FDA can take court action to remove the products of concern. The need to recall a product is identified through any information that indicates a potential defect posing a health risk. Examples of this include reports of adverse events associated with a specific lot, or a problem noted with a piece of equipment used in manufacturing that may have been defective while preparing previously released lots. When a recall is submitted, the FDA completes an evaluation to assign a recall classification of Class I – III with Class I having reasonable probability of serious health consequences or death due to the use of the drug and Class III being unlikely to cause health consequences [46]. The evaluation points used by the FDA to determine the recall class include the following:

– if disease or other injuries have already occurred from use of the drug
– if existing conditions could lead to a human or animal health hazard
– the degree of seriousness of the hazard
– the significance of the consequences of the hazard

Based on this evaluation, a recall level will be determined. The potential recall levels are consumer/user level, retail level, or wholesale level [46]. In the case of a recalled drug, the wholesale level would be contacting wholesalers with the recall information to remove all of their stock. The retail level would involve contacting the distributors that have purchased the product through wholesalers or direct from the manufacturer so that unsold product can be returned. In the case of drugs, this would be veterinarians and pharmacies being contacted. Recall to the consumer/ user level would involve contacting individual clients that have purchased the product.

When a recall is requested, the firm requesting it will develop a recall strategy that considers the specifics of the situation with this plan being reviewed by the FDA prior to implementation [46]. Depending on the severity of the recall, public notice may be provided by press releases. A searchable database of recalls can be found on the FDA's Recalls, Market Withdrawals, & Safety Alerts page. Additional information about safety of drugs can be found on FDA's MedWatch page for human drugs and on FDA's Animal & Veterinary Recalls & Withdrawals page for animal drugs. Compounding pharmacy recalls can be found on FDA's Compounding: Inspections, Recalls, and other Actions page, which covers human compounding, but some pharmacies may also prepare compounds for animal patients. An additional FDA webpage, Inspections, Recalls, and Other Actions with Respect to Firms that Engage in Animal Drug Compounding, pulls out pharmacies that are known to prepare compounds for animal patients.

If you received notice that a product has been recalled, check your stock, and remove any of the specified lots. Follow the directions on the recall notification with regard to returning the affected lots and any additional notification that is recommended. Document the actions taken on the request form and file for your records.

Selecting a Compounding Pharmacy

When humans are involved, errors will occur. Therefore, all the problems discussed in this chapter could potentially occur at any compounding pharmacy. That is why there are USP chapters describing minimum best practices and cGMP standards for outsourcing facilities manufacturing large quantities of compounded medications. The intent is that there are enough checks and balances in place to ensure that errors are difficult to make, and if they do occur, they are caught prior to the medication reaching a patient. However, this is not foolproof as oversight through inspection is state dependent and often sporadic. There is also clinical judgment through the knowledge of formulation development and veterinary pharmacy specifics that can impact the quality and appropriateness of a compound. Therefore, it is important to critically evaluate the compounding pharmacies you send prescriptions to. Chapter 4 will discuss compounding pharmacy selection in more detail.

Client Education

An important component of the risk–benefit analysis of compounded medications is client education. The human version of client education is patient counseling. This is required by all state pharmacy acts at least for new prescriptions unless the patient or their representative declines. Therefore, patient counseling will occur when medications come from human pharmacies. If you have ever picked up a new prescription medication from a pharmacy, you have experienced a form of patient counseling, which may have been limited to the person checking you out asking if you have any questions for the pharmacist and documenting that you declined when you said you did not have questions. If you did have questions, the pharmacist was likely happy to address those. However, even if our clients have questions when picking up their pet's medications, the pharmacist may not have sufficient resources or education to fully address those questions. That is where it falls to the veterinarian to ensure that clients leave with an appropriate level of education about the medications being prescribed.

Providing this client education about compounded medications provides several benefits. First, it provides an opportunity to discuss with the client the fact that you are prescribing a compounded medication instead of a commercial product and why. The general public may have heard of compounding from the media, but they usually lack a full understanding of the difference between compounded and approved medications. Common misconceptions are that compounded medications are the same as generic medications or the opposite end of the spectrum that compounded medications are ineffective and potentially dangerous. Therefore, it is important to identify a client's current knowledge of/experience with compounded medications and further educate from there. This education also ties in well to discussing the risks versus benefits of compounds in general as well as the specific one you are prescribing. You likely considered all the points in this chapter and conducted a risk–benefit analysis in your head in the span of a few minutes or less. However, you will need to summarize this to bring the client up to speed. Since not all sources of compounded medications are the same, you will want to address with the client whether this is a medication you can provide from the clinic and/or what compounding pharmacy you recommend they obtain it from.

When providing this information to a client, it may be overwhelming for them to digest depending on how much other information was provided to them and their healthcare literacy. Therefore, handouts can be helpful to provide. One option is to have a standard form handout for your practice that states that a compounded medication is being prescribed, lists the general risks of compounded medications, and then leaves a place for adding in the specific reasons why the benefits of the compound you are prescribing outweigh these risks.

Reducing Risk in Practice

This chapter discussed a lot of risks as well as examples that these problems are actually occurring and are not only theoretical. However, this chapter also highlighted the reasons why we frequently need to reach for compounded medications. A common concern is what is the legal liability of the veterinarian if the pharmacy provides an incorrect compound and harm occurs. The answer to this is not clear, but comprehensive documentation of why the compound was necessary as well as the client education that was provided can help decrease liability. The authors recommend engaging legal counsel to develop a comprehensive strategy to decrease your liability. However, the following suggestions provide a basic good documentation foundation.

1) Document in the patient record the reason for prescribing the compounded medication. If the reason is client-based (e.g. ease of administration), the rationale should also include the mention of any discussion that was had with the client about ability to administer the approved version.

2) Develop a standard client handout template for all the compounded medications prescribed and make it practice policy that this is provided each time a compounded medication is prescribed. Consider whether the client should sign to indicate that they have received this information and agree with the plan to utilize a compounded medication.

3) Ensure that client education and documentation policies are consistently followed by all the doctors in the practice.

4) Critically evaluate compounding pharmacies to create a list of a few pharmacies that appear to be high quality and can provide the compounded medications utilized in your patient population. See Chapter 4 for additional details on compounding pharmacy evaluation.

5) Ask clients to contact the clinic if any potential adverse effects or signs of quality problems are noted. When contacted by clients, ensure that the adverse effects and quality problems are reported appropriately.

6) When requesting new/less common formulations of a drug, ask the pharmacist what data they have available to support its efficacy and stability. All too often pharmacists assume that if a veterinarian is requesting a formulation, it must work, and veterinarians assume that if a pharmacist agrees to make a formulation, it must work, which results in no one critically evaluating the appropriateness of a formulation. The best outcomes will occur when pharmacists and veterinarians work together to determine the appropriateness of a formulation.

Conclusion

Veterinary medicine is full of trade-offs. For example, the gold standard treatment often comes at a higher cost. The utilization of compounded medications is another example of the risk–benefit analysis that we incorporate into patient care. While the benefits of compounded medications are widely understood, the risks are often less so, especially for our clients. The information in this chapter was designed to provide background on those risks as well as risk mitigation strategies that are in place and the gaps inherently present in those. Future chapters will provide additional insight into topics that can assist with risk reduction.

References

1 Compounding FAQ for veterinarians. American Veterinary Medical Association. https://www.avma.org/resources-tools/animal-health-and-welfare/animal-health/compounding/compounding-faq-veterinarians (accessed 22 September 2022).

2 Sartor, L.L., Trepanier, L.A., Kroll, M.M. et al. (2004). Efficacy and safety of transdermal methimazole in the treatment of cats with hyperthyroidism. *J. Vet. Intern. Med.* 18 (5): https://doi.org/10.1892/0891-6640(2004)18<651:EASOTM>2.0.CO;2.

3 Li, X., Li, W., Wang, H. et al. (2006). Cats lack a sweet taste receptor. *J. Nutr.* 136 (7): 1932S–1934S. https://doi.org/10.1093/jn/136.7.1932S.

4 USP (2019). *USP General Chapter <795> Pharmaceutical Compounding – Nonsterile Preparations*. Rockville, MD: USP.

5 (2020). Piroxicam – Plumb's veterinary drugs. https://app.plumbs.com/drug-monograph/mbT3Y ecrKAPROD?section=doses&source=search&searchQuery=piroxicam (accessed 22 September 2022).

6 Piroxicam. https://doi.usp.org/USPNF/USPNF_M65720_05_01.html (accessed 22 September 2022.)

7 Murphy, L.A. and Coleman, A.E. (2012). Xylitol toxicosis in dogs. *Vet. Clin. North Am. Small Anim. Pract.* 42 (2): 307–312. https://doi.org/10.1016/j.cvsm.2011.12.003.

8 Peterson, M.E. (2013). Xylitol. *Top. Companion Anim. Med.* 28 (1): 18–20. https://doi.org/10.1053/j.tcam.2013.03.008.

9 Paws off! Xylitol is toxic to dogs. FDA. https://www.fda.gov/animal-veterinary/animal-health-literacy/paws-xylitol-toxic-dogs (accessed 22 September 2022).

10 eCFR :: 21 CFR part 530 -- extralabel drug use in animals. https://www.ecfr.gov/current/title-21/part-530 (accessed 22 September 2022).

11 Animal Medicinal Drug Use Clarification Act (AMDUCA). American Veterinary Medical Association. https://www.avma.org/resources-tools/animal-health-and-welfare/amduca (accessed 22 September 2022).

12 (2010). U.S.C. Title 21 – food and drugs. https://www.govinfo.gov/content/pkg/USCODE-2010-title21/html/USCODE-2010-title21-chap9-subchapII.htm (accessed 22 September 2022).

13 (2020). From an idea to the marketplace: the journey of an animal drug through the approval process. FDA. https://www.fda.gov/animal-veterinary/animal-health-literacy/idea-marketplace-journey-animal-drug-through-approval-process (accessed 22 September 2022).

14 (2022). Approval and Regulation of Animal Medicines. Animal Health Institute. https://ahi.org/approval-and-regulation-of-animal-medicines (accessed 22 September 2022).

15 Rockville (2018). *United States Pharmacopeia (USP 41. NF – 36)*.

16 (2022). CFR – Code of Federal Regulations title 21. https://www.accessdata.fda.gov/scripts/cdrh/cfdocs/cfcfr/CFRSearch.cfm?CFRPart=211 (accessed 22 September 2022).

17 Umstead, M.E., Boothe, D.M., Cruz-Espindola, C. et al. (2012). Accuracy and precision of compounded ciclosporin capsules and solution. *Vet. Dermatol.* 23 (5): https://doi.org/10.1111/j.1365-3164.2012.01078.x.

18 Thompson, J.A., Mirza, M.H., Barker, S.A. et al. (2011). Clenbuterol toxicosis in three quarter horse racehorses after administration of a compounded product. *J. Am. Vet. Med. Assoc.* 239 (6): https://doi.org/10.2460/javma.239.6.842.

19 McConkey, S.E., Walker, S., and Adams, C. (2012). Compounding errors in 2 dogs receiving anticonvulsants. *Can. Vet. J.* 53 (4): 391–394.

20 Robat, C. and Budde, J. (2017). Potency and stability of compounded cyclophosphamide: a pilot study. *Vet. Comp. Oncol.* 15 (3): https://doi.org/10.1111/vco.12210.

21 Burton, J.H., Knych, H.K., Stanley, S.D., and Rebhun, R.B. (2017). Potency and stability of compounded formulations of chlorambucil, melphalan and cyclophosphamide. *Vet. Comp. Oncol.* 15 (4): https://doi.org/10.1111/vco.12301.

22 Burton, J.H., Stanley, S.D., Knych, H.K. et al. (2016). Frequency and severity of neutropenia associated with Food and Drug Administration approved and compounded formulations of lomustine in dogs with cancer. *J. Vet. Intern. Med.* 30 (1): https://doi.org/10.1111/jvim.13805.

23 KuKanich, B., Warner, M., and Hahn, K. (2017). Analysis of lomustine drug content in FDA-approved and compounded lomustine capsules. *J. Am. Vet. Med. Assoc.* 250 (3): https://doi.org/10.2460/javma.250.3.322.

24 Johnson, L.R., Weaver, P.G., Forsythe, L.E. et al. (2021). Drug content on receipt and over time for compounded formulations of famciclovir. *J. Feline Med. Surg.* 23 (6): https://doi.org/10.1177/1098612X20961046.

25 O'Leary, L.M., Allbaugh, R.A., Schrunk, D.E. et al. (2021). Variable accuracy, precision, and consistency of compounded famciclovir formulated for management of feline herpesvirus-1 in cats. *Vet. Ophthalmol.* 24 (6): https://doi.org/10.1111/vop.12910.

26 KuKanich, K., KuKanich, B., Slead, T., and Warner, M. (2017). Evaluation of drug content (potency) for compounded and FDA–approved formulations of doxycycline on receipt and after 21 days of storage. *J. Am. Vet. Med. Assoc.* 251 (7): 835–842. https://doi.org/10.2460/javma.251.7.835.

27 Laporte, C.M., Cruz-Espindola, C., Thungrat, K. et al. (2017). Quality assessment of fluconazole capsules and oral suspensions compounded by pharmacies located in the United States. *Am. J. Vet. Res.* 78 (4): 421–432. https://doi.org/10.2460/ajvr.78.4.421.

28 Scott-Moncrieff, J.C.R., Moore, G.E., Coe, J. et al. (2012). Characteristics of commercially manufactured and compounded protamine zinc insulin. *J. Am. Vet. Med. Assoc.* 240 (5): 600–605. https://doi.org/10.2460/javma.240.5.600.

29 Stanley, S.D., Thomasy, S.M., and Skinner, W. (2003). Comparison for pharmaceutical equivalence of FDA-approved products and compounded preparations of Ketoprofen, Amikacin, and Boldenone. IVIS. https://www.ivis.org/library/aaep/aaep-annual-convention-new-orleans-2003/comparison-for-pharmaceutical-equivalence-of (accessed 22 September 2022).

30 Cook, A.K., Nieuwoudt, C.D., and Longhofer, S.L. (2012). Pharmaceutical evaluation of compounded trilostane products. *J. Am. Anim. Hosp. Assoc.* 48 (4): 228–233. https://doi.org/10.5326/JAAHA-MS-5763.

31 Shah, M., Sandler, L., Rai, V. et al. (2013). Quality of compounded topical 2% diltiazem hydrochloride formulations for anal fissure. *World J. Gastroenterol.* 19 (34): https://doi.org/10.3748/wjg.v19.i34.5645.

32 Meyer, L.M., Stephens, K., Carter, C.A. et al. (2020). Stability and consistency of compounded oral liquid levothyroxine formulations. *J. Am. Pharm. Assoc.* 60 (6): https://doi.org/10.1016/j.japh.2020.05.014.

33 Papich, M.G., Davidson, G.S., and Fortier, L.A. (2013). Doxycycline concentration over time after storage in a compounded veterinary preparation. *J. Am. Vet. Med. Assoc.* 242 (12): https://doi.org/10.2460/javma.242.12.1674.

34 Boulton, D.W., Paul Fawcett, J., and Woods, D.J. (1996). Stability of an extemporaneously compounded levothyroxine sodium oral liquid. *Am. J. Health Syst. Pharm.* 53 (10): 1157–1161. https://doi.org/10.1093/ajhp/53.10.1157.

35 Molter, C.M., Zuba, J.R., and Papendick, R. (2014). *Cryptococcus gattii* osteomyelitis and compounded itraconazole treatment failure in a Pesquet's parrot (*Psittrichas fulgidus*). *J. Zoo Wildl. Med.* 45 (1): 127–133. https://doi.org/10.1638/2013-0042R1.1.

36 Smith, J.A., Papich, M.G., Russell, G., and Mitchell, M.A. (2010). Effects of compounding on pharmacokinetics of itraconazole in black-footed penguins (*Spheniscus demersus*). *J. Zoo Wildl. Med.* 41 (3): https://doi.org/10.1638/2010-0019.1.

37 Mawby, D.I., Whittemore, J.C., Fowler, L.E., and Papich, M.G. (2018). Comparison of absorption characteristics of oral reference and compounded itraconazole formulations in healthy cats. *J. Am. Vet. Med. Assoc.* 252 (2): https://doi.org/10.2460/javma.252.2.195.

38 Mawby, D.I., Whittemore, J.C., Genger, S., and Papich, M.G. (2014). Bioequivalence of orally administered generic, compounded, and innovator-formulated itraconazole in healthy dogs. *J. Vet. Intern. Med.* 28 (1): https://doi.org/10.1111/jvim.12219.

39 Merritt, A.M., Sanchez, L.C., Burrow, J.A. et al. (2003). Effect of GastroGard and three compounded oral omeprazole preparations on 24 h intragastric pH in gastrically cannulated mature horses. *Equine Vet. J.* 35 (7): https://doi.org/10.2746/042516403775696339.

40 Nieto, J.E., Spier, S., Pipers, F.S. et al. (2002). Comparison of paste and suspension formulations of omeprazole in the healing of gastric ulcers in racehorses in active training. *J. Am. Vet. Med. Assoc.* 221 (8): https://doi.org/10.2460/javma.2002.221.1139.

41 Trissel, L.A., Gentempo, J.A., Anderson, R.W., and Lajeunesse, J.D. (2005). Using a medium-fill simulation to evaluate the microbial contamination rate for USP medium-risk-level compounding. *Am. J. Health Syst. Pharm.* 62 (3): https://doi.org/10.1093/ajhp/62.3.285.

42 Stucki, C., Sautter, A.M., Favet, J., and Bonnabry, P. (2009). Microbial contamination of syringes during preparation: the direct influence of environmental cleanliness and risk manipulations on end-product quality. *Am. J. Health Syst. Pharm.* 66 (22): https://doi.org/10.2146/ajhp070681.

43 Power, L.A., Coyne, J.W., and Hawkins, B. (2018). ASHP guidelines on handling hazardous drugs. *Am. J. Health Syst. Pharm.* 75 (24): https://doi.org/10.2146/ajhp180564.

44 (2022). How to report animal drug and device side effects and product problems. FDA. https://www.fda.gov/animal-veterinary/report-problem/how-report-animal-drug-and-device-side-effects-and-product-problems (accessed 22 September 2022).

45 (2022). Adverse event reports for animal drugs and devices. FDA. https://www.fda.gov/animal-veterinary/product-safety-information/adverse-event-reports-animal-drugs-and-devices (accessed 22 September 2022).

46 (2022). CFR – Code of Federal Regulations title 21. https://www.accessdata.fda.gov/scripts/cdrh/cfdocs/cfcfr/CFRSearch.cfm?CFRPart=7 (accessed 22 September 2022).

3

Beyond-Use Dating

Determining an effective beyond-use date (BUD) is a critical component of both sterile and nonsterile compounding as it indicates the date and time after which a compound must not be used. BUDs are calculated from the date/time that the compound was prepared. They are similar to expiration dates in that the medication must not be administered after that date. Both BUDs and expiration dates are determined based on when a medication will degrade to the point that it contains active drug or toxin levels outside of ranges allowed in official compendia. These dates also take into consideration potential microbial growth that may affect the preparation. A major difference between BUDs and expiration dates is the amount of data used to support the dating. BUDs are often determined based on significantly less robust data than that used for establishing expiration dates. This is appropriate when considered in the context that compounding is designed to be unique, patient-specific preparations made in accordance with a prescription, so the several-year shelf life seen with manufactured products is not necessary or appropriate. For that reason, BUDs are often much shorter than the expiration date of a manufactured product. The following sections will review the factors affecting BUDs, how to identify appropriate studies for extending BUDs, and considerations when evaluating the BUDs on compounded medications prepared by outside pharmacies. Chapter 5 will discuss the methods for determining BUDs for formulations compounded in-house in more depth.

Factors Considered When Assigning BUDs and Expiration Dates

BUDs and expiration dates both indicate the time after which a drug must not be used. Using a drug after the stated BUD or expiration date would constitute the use of an adulterated drug that is prohibited in the Food, Drug, and Cosmetic (FD&C) Act. Per the FD&C Act, "a drug shall be deemed to be adulterated if the methods used in, or the facilities or controls used for its manufacturer, processing, packing, or holding do not conform to or are not operated or administered in conformity with current good manufacturing practice to assure that such drug meets the requirement of the act as to safety and has the identity and strength, and meets the quality and purity characteristics, which it purports or is represented to possess" [1]. Both expiration and BUDs are determined based on the type of drug and its mechanism(s) of degradation, the dosage form and additional ingredients, the likelihood that microbial growth will occur, the packaging of the final

Drug Compounding for Veterinary Professionals, First Edition. Lauren R. Eichstadt Forsythe and Alexandria E. Gochenauer.
© 2023 John Wiley & Sons, Inc. Published 2023 by John Wiley & Sons, Inc.
Companion Website: www.wiley.com/go/forsythe/drug

dosage form, and expected storage conditions. The evaluation of stability includes physical stability, chemical stability, and performance over time [2].

Manufactured products (including 503b compounds) must adhere to CFR Part 211 when assigning expiration dates. If a manufactured product is a powder requiring reconstitution, the expiration date requirements must be applied to identify expiration dates for the powder form as well as the liquid after reconstitution. Stability testing with validated stability-indicating methods must be used for determining the expiration dates of manufactured products. This testing must be done on several batches of product and based on storage in the same container-closure system that will be used for the final product. CFR Part 211 does allow for the use of accelerated studies in combination with basic stability information on the drug, excipients, and container-closure system to establish a tentative expiration date while full shelf-life studies are being conducted [3].

The United States Pharmacopeia (USP) defines stability as "the extent to which a product retains, within specified limits, and throughout its period of storage and use (i.e. its shelf life), the same properties and characteristics that it possessed at the time of its manufacture" [4]. The evaluation of stability includes physical, chemical, microbiological, therapeutic, and toxicological. The USP defines physical stability as "the ability of a material to remain physically unchanged over time under stated or reasonably expected conditions for manufacturing, storage, and use" [5]. This includes palatability, appearance, dissolution, uniformity, and ability to be resuspended. Physical stability requires that product physical changes, such as drug separation/settling, must be easily reversed. An example of this would be shaking a suspension to redisperse the drug that has settled. If the drug can be easily redispersed with shaking, that is an acceptable physical change. However, if the drug has caked to the bottom of the container and is not redistributable, then that may indicate a lack of physical stability. Physical stability can be affected by a variety of forces, including light, pH, temperature, and humidity.

Chemical stability requires that all the active ingredients maintain their chemical integrity and labeled potency. Differentiating between physical and chemical instability can be difficult. For example, a color change may reflect a chemical or physical change, or oxidation, which is a chemical event, may trigger aggregation, which is a physical change [5]. However, whether the degradation is physical or chemical is not critical to determine from the perspective of compounding. Regardless of the type of degradation, BUDs and expiration dates are determined to ensure that the use of the product does not continue past the point of clinically significant degradation. Processes that are likely to cause drug degradation without a visual or scent change are hydrolysis, epimerization, decarboxylation, dehydration, oxidation, photochemical decomposition, ionic strength, pH, interionic compatibility issues, and temperature [4]. Which degradation mechanisms apply to a particular drug is somewhat predictable. For example, esters, such as lidocaine and bupivacaine, and beta-lactams are most likely to hydrolyze when water is present, and epinephrine and other catecholamines are likely to oxidize. Knowing what drugs or drug classes experience which degradation mechanisms allow manufacturers to prepare products in such a way as to delay degradation as much as possible. In these examples, beta-lactam liquids can be reconstituted immediately prior to use and hydrolysis can be slowed by storage at refrigerated temperatures, and epinephrine can be packed into vials/ampules in a nitrogen atmosphere to prevent oxidation. Some of these techniques, such as refrigerated storage, can be used to increase compound stability, but others like the nitrogen atmosphere are much more difficult and costly to implement at a compounding scale.

When considering the stability of compounds, it is important to keep in mind that formulation changes that change the ionic strength or the pH of the solution/suspension [3] can significantly increase the rate of drug degradation. An approved drug solution that is stable for an extended period may degrade quickly when mixed with another drug or excipient that changes the pH. A single-unit pH change has the potential to decrease drug stability by 10 times or more [4]. Often, a pH buffer system is used as an excipient in liquid preparations to maintain the pH within the range where the drug is most stable. pH is one example of the significant effect excipients can have on formulations and why when using extended stability studies, it is critical that the formulation being made is identical to the studied formulation. Excipients affecting stability is one example of how a compounded drug prepared at one pharmacy may have different stability than the same drug prepared at a different pharmacy.

With regard to temperature, it is generally assumed that the rate of a chemical reaction occurring such as hydrolysis or oxidation increases exponentially for each $10\,°C$ temperature increase. For example, if a beta-lactam antibiotic suspension is stored at room temperature, it can be expected that the shelf life will decrease to $\frac{1}{4}$ to $\frac{1}{25}$ of the refrigerated shelf life. While colder temperatures can have a positive effect on stability, there is also a potential for negative effects. For example, increased viscosity for some refrigerated liquids and thawing of frozen emulsions can cause stability problems, so a blanket assumption that refrigerated or frozen products have significantly increased stability is not appropriate [4].

Microbiological, therapeutic, and toxicological stabilities are markers of performance stability. These require that the product maintains sterility or resistance to microbial growth based on formulation requirements and its therapeutic effect without any significant increase in toxicity. Like physical and chemical stability can blend into each other, performance stability parameters are closely related to physical and chemical stability. If a product has limited chemical stability, it is likely that the therapeutic and/or toxicological stability will be negatively impacted due to the degradation of the active ingredient(s) and/or the increase in toxic products of degradation.

Many stability issues can only be identified through specific testing. However, some changes can be seen with a visual evaluation of a product, making the visual examination of a product an important component of compound quality. A few examples of visual stability issues are listed below [5], and Figure 3.1 shows an example of visually unstable otic suspensions.

– Tablets with visible crumbling may indicate water sorption.
– A solution that has turned hazy can indicate microbial growth or drug degradation that lead to a precipitate.
– A viscosity change in an ointment may indicate the recrystallization of a drug.

While determining exactly how long a drug product is good for requires validated method stability-indicating studies of the exact formulation under the actual storage conditions including the same container-closure system, there are certain characteristics that indicate that a drug may be more susceptible to degradation. The following are some potential characteristics that increase the likelihood a drug will degrade quickly [5]. These should be taken into consideration when determining if a USP default BUD is appropriate for the specific drug and formulation.

– Low-melting-point drugs may be more likely to experience phase changes.
– For combination products or excipient combinations, mixing acids and bases can increase the likelihood that salts will form.
– Hygroscopic drugs and excipients are more likely to absorb moisture from the environment leading to physical changes.

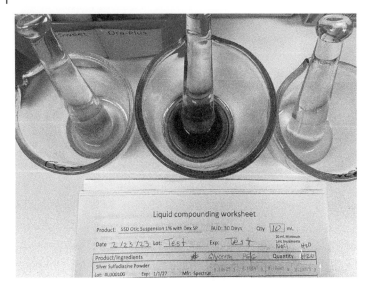

Figure 3.1 An SSD + Dexamethasone SP otic solution compound made in three different vehicles. The left formulation utilized bacteriostatic water, the center formulation utilized bacteriostatic saline, and the right formulation utilized anhydrous glycerin. The color changes seen with the left and center formulations indicate a stability concern likely due to the SSD interacting with the preservative and the sodium chloride components.

- Preparation techniques, such as stirring and milling, heating, and cooling, and high-heat terminal sterilization can lead to stability problems.
- Poor temperature and/or humidity control in preparation, and ingredient or finished product storage areas can lead to physical instability.

USP Default BUDs

Compounded products prepared in 503a facilities that utilize USP compounding standards have BUDs assigned to them instead of expiration dates. While still used to indicate the time after which a product must not be used, BUD terminology is used to distinguish this dating from an expiration date. Since compounded medications are intended for immediate or short-term administration pursuant to a prescription, the dating is established with that in mind. BUDs are determined based on hours, days, or months with a maximum BUD of 180 days due to the patient-specific intent of the use of compounded medications.

The USP establishes these default BUDs in General Chapters 795 and 797 for nonsterile and sterile compounded preparations, respectively. These default BUDs address the need for a standard for BUDs for compounds when the full studies conducted on manufactured products are not feasible. These dates are science-based estimates of a timeframe for which most formulations with a set of similar characteristics are expected to meet compendial standards. The USP default BUDs create general groups of compounds based on characteristics that are likely to affect stability over days to months. These are primarily based on water activity (aqueous versus nonaqueous), storage temperature, the presence of a preservative, and, for sterile compounds, the environment in which the compound is prepared. The USP also allows the extension of BUDs based on product-specific studies and the shortening of the default BUDs based on studies or professional judgment indicating that the specific formulation is likely to degrade before the default BUD is reached.

Stability Studies

As the above information describes, determining the stability of a compounded medication is complicated and impractical to do for every individualized medication needed. Therefore, the USP provides default BUDs that can be used for compounded medications in lieu of full studies such as those conducted for manufactured products. These BUDs are based on a timeframe where it is likely that a drug meeting the specified characteristics will maintain its stability. The USP also allows for extending the BUD beyond the default based on stability-indicating studies. USP default dates are often short for many oral products, thus increasing the burden on the client, pharmacy, and veterinarian to obtain small amounts frequently. Therefore, it is desirable to use extended stability data to lengthen the BUD. Even for compounds that have sufficiently long default BUDs, stability studies can support the default date for a formulation of a drug that is known to be frequently unstable, such as doxycycline liquid compounds, or indicate that dating shorter than the USP default is necessary.

Since product BUDs have a significant impact on the practicality and cost of a compounded medication, stability studies are frequently published, referenced, and/or conducted internally. That said, not all studies reporting the stability of a compound are created equal or are sufficient for extending the BUD beyond the USP default. Studying product stability has been occurring since the 1950s, and several articles/editorials were authored by Lawrence Trissel in the 1980s explaining the characteristics of a reliable stability study. These articles described five areas where published stability studies frequently fell short [6–8]. The five points described by Trissel in 1983 and summarized below remain helpful today when evaluating stability studies to determine their appropriateness for extending BUDs.

1) The description of the materials, methods, and test conditions must be sufficiently detailed to allow the replication of the study. Small changes in temperature, concentration, the presence/absence of light, storage container, and ingredients can have a significant effect on drug stability. If a study found that a drug degraded by 15% within 12 hours without indicating the storage temperature, that study has questionable relevance until you know the storage temperature. It cannot be concluded that this same result would be seen at all temperatures. Could refrigerated storage slow the drug degradation or was this the degradation observed with refrigerated storage? Without the details of the temperature used in the study, clinical application is not feasible. Similarly, the exact ingredients used must be described. Similar products from different manufacturers may have differing formulations that affect stability. Without the details of which manufacturer was used for each ingredient, it becomes difficult to replicate the formulation in practice. It is also critical that the concentrations of the compound tested are disclosed. A combination that is stable at a low concentration may not be stable at a higher concentration.

2) The assay used must be stability-indicating. For an assay to be stability-indicating, it must detect and separate the intact drug from all decomposition products, other drugs, and other components of the solution. If the study fails to prove that the method used is stability-indicating, the results are suspect at best because decomposition products may be interfering with the test. Stability-indicating assays are often accomplished using high-performance liquid chromatography (HPLC) but could also be done using radioimmunoassay, enzyme-multiplied immunoassay technique, enzyme-linked immunosorbent assay, or a fluorescence polarization immunoassay (TDX). While all of these can be stability-indicating, they are not always stability-indicating. Therefore, all of these must include validation that the method used is stability-indicating for

the specific drug being evaluated. Example methods of validation include subjecting the fresh, intact drug to severe stress such as intensive heating and pH extremes, or mixing a solution of intact drug with known decomposition products. After one of these manipulations, the resulting solution is analyzed to determine if the drug is selectively detected versus all of the decomposition products and other components.

A study by Ray et al. [9] provides an example of problems that may occur when an assay is not validated as stability-indicating. This study described an HPLC method to determine the stability of tetrahydrocannabinol (THC) capsules, which produced a peak neatly separated from known degradation products. However, when stored under high-temperature conditions, the THC peak width increased slightly. This width increase was determined to be an unresolved peak with the THC and a degradation product eluting together. The result was that the capsules appeared more stable than they actually were. Immunoassays are also susceptible to problems when the validation of the stability-indicating nature is not done. In this case, incorrect results may occur due to the antibody binding with related chemical entities that are degradants similar in structure to the active drug.

3) The study must determine the actual drug concentration at time-zero. There are several factors described in Chapter 2 that can result in an actual concentration that differs from the target concentration. It is realistic to assume that these variables may result in a starting concentration that is 80–120% of the target concentration [7]. Therefore, without having the initial concentration, the study cannot produce accurate conclusions. For example, a study may find that at the first study time-point of four hours, the concentration is 88% of the target concentration, therefore concluding that the drug degraded by 12% in four hours. However, if the starting concentration was only 90% of the target concentration, this creates a different interpretation of the stability.

4) The study should utilize replicate assays. By testing replicate solutions, the study authors minimize the impact of human error and assay variability and are more likely to identify erroneous outliers. There is no specific rule about how many tests and samples must be used. However, it is generally considered appropriate if a study uses duplicate assays of three replicate test solutions.

5) The conclusions must fit the actual results obtained. Stability and compatibility are always relative. Therefore, stability studies often require conclusions with several qualifiers due to the significant effect small variations may have on stability and compatibility. It is important that the conclusions are only as definitive as the results support and that all results are considered, even those that are considered inconvenient or not easily explained. For example, a study that is looking at the stability of a solution of Drug A and Drug B with a method that is only proven to be stability-indicating for Drug A cannot conclude anything about the stability of Drug B. The conclusions should simply state the conclusion for Drug A in the presence of B and that the stability of Drug B was not evaluated.

Evaluating Stability Studies

Although the above stability study requirements were published in the 1980s, there is still an accumulated body of stability studies that do not comply. Trissel noted that between the initial description of these five major requirements in 1983 and a follow-up editorial in 1988, there was significant improvement in manuscripts that effectively met the criteria except for the requirement to report a validated stability-indicating method. Trissel noted that the argument is not with the premise but rather with the proof [8]. The validation of the method adds an additional step to the drug analysis, which significantly increases the cost of having these studies completed. Therefore, there is a temptation for compounds to be evaluated using a "potency over time" model where nonstability indicating methods appropriate at time-zero are used repeatedly over an extended period in an attempt to support extended stability. However, as described above, conclusions drawn from this are unreliable, making it an inappropriate method.

Stability studies can be found in a wide variety of veterinary and human medical journals with increased density in journals that frequently publish pharmacology topics. Since the 1980s, progressively fewer studies with inadequate or nonexistent validation of the stability-indicating capability are making it into the literature. However, there are still enough studies that were previously published to warrant a critical evaluation of stability studies used for extended beyond-use dating. It is also important to consider that USP default BUDs can be extended based on unpublished stability data, so it is prudent to ensure that a pharmacy that is utilizing unpublished data for a competitive advantage is using validated stability-indicating methods.

Evaluating whether a stability study is stability-indicating does not require extensive knowledge of analytical techniques. As a clinician, there are a few key things that you can look for. When describing the stability-indicating validation, the authors may either reference another validated method if noted that it was used exactly as previously described or document their own validation. To conduct their own validation, they can either subject the fresh, intact drug to severe stress such as intensive heating and pH extremes or mix a solution of intact drug with known decomposition products. If their analytical method can selectively detect drug versus all other components and decomposition products, then it is stability-indicating [7]. Key words often found in studies that have conducted this evaluation include "stability-indicating," and/or "forced degradation." This level of detail may or may not appear in the abstract, so a review of the analytical methods section may be required. If it cannot be determined that a study used a validated stability-indicating method, then the results are unreliable, and the study is not sufficient for extending the BUD beyond USP defaults.

Determining BUDs for In-House Formulations

When developing nonsterile formulations to compound in-house, there are a few options for establishing the BUD. These includes utilizing USP default dates, referencing a USP monograph, and referencing published stability studies. Below is a summary of each with more details provided in Chapter 5.

USP default dates for nonsterile compounds are provided in the current version of USP General Chapter 795. These dates are conservative and represent a timeframe that the majority of drugs meeting the specified characteristics will remain stable. The default date for the formulation type in question is an appropriate BUD to use when a published stability study or USP monograph is not available for the exact formulation being studied. However, if available data indicates concerns that the formulation will remain stable for the default BUD, then a shorter BUD must be used. If using one of the following methods to support extended dating, ensure that all requirements in the current version of applicable USP chapters are addressed.

USP monographs are available for a wide variety of compounds. Some of these are compounds specifically identified for veterinary use (e.g. enrofloxacin), while others may be used for human or veterinary use. These compound monographs provide a description of the formulation preparation and storage as well as the determined stability. The authors recommend using a USP monograph for establishing a BUD if possible as these are all stability-indicating studies that clearly provide the information needed to create a master formulation and meet the USP requirements for extending the BUD.

Published stability studies that meet the quality criteria described earlier in this chapter can be referenced on the master formulation to support an extended BUD. However, it is important to ensure that the formulation being prepared is identical to the formulation studied. One exception to this is bracketing of the concentration. If there are two studies supporting extended stability of the same formulation differing only in concentration, then any concentration falling between the two studied can be considered stable for the duration reported in the studies. For example, if stability studies are available showing three-month stability of Drug A at 1 and 10 mg/ml prepared and stored in an identical manner, then these studies can be referenced to support a three-month BUD for Drug A at 5 mg/ml prepared and stored in the same manner as the studies. This concept also applies to USP monographs.

BUD Considerations When Prescribing Compounded Medications

When prescribing compounded medications, it is important to keep BUD in mind both with respect to the duration of therapy prescribed as well as drug integrity. If a particular compound is only going to have a 30-day BUD, then it is not practical to prescribe a 60-day supply. This can be remedied by prescribing the 30-day supply with refills. For products with BUDs that are less than the duration a client may wish to obtain, it is important to make the client aware of the reason for the decreased supply. The amount that can be prescribed for products with a short BUD will also be affected if the medication is being shipped and the client needs to request a refill far enough in advance to have it on hand when running out. Consider this example. An oral suspension has a BUD of 30 days from the day it is compounded. The patient will need 18 ml of solution for a 30-day supply of the medication. To provide a bit of cushion for drug loss, you prescribe 20 ml for a 30-day supply with three refills. This medication is coming from a compounding pharmacy that will ship the medication to the client with overnight shipping being significantly more expensive than regular shipping. The first time, the client gets the medication two days after you prescribe it and starts therapy. At this point, two days of the 30-day time period have passed, meaning that the client will likely have about two more days of medication left when it reaches the BUD. They plan proactively and call for a refill a couple of days before their current bottle expires. The refill is requested on a Thursday morning, and the current bottle is good through Sunday. Since the first bottle came in two days with standard shipping, they opt for that again. The medication is prepared on Thursday and shipped that day and gets to the client on Saturday. They use the original bottle on Sunday and then discard and start the new bottle on Monday. At this point, the new bottle is now on the fifth day of 30 before it expires despite getting the same 20 ml originally prescribed. This problem is likely to continue for subsequent fills. This is the point where clients often get frustrated that they are paying for shipping monthly and not even getting a full month out of the bottle before it expires. Depending on the medication, this would be a case to consider a local compounding pharmacy and/or the feasibility of preparing the compounded medication in-house.

The temptation in the above example may be to tell the client that it is okay to use the compound for an extra couple of days beyond the BUD since it is often not an exact date anyway. However, this is not a legal or clinically advisable recommendation. Pharmacies generally use the longest BUD possible for a compound because it helps both client satisfaction and their workflow. Therefore, when a pharmacy has a compound with a short BUD, it is reasonable to assume that is the longest date that can legally and/or clinically be applied based on the information available to them. Even if the date is a USP default BUD that is likely conservative, recall that the FD&C Act states a drug is adulterated, and therefore, it is illegal to use/recommend its use once it passes the expiration date or BUD.

In addition to the considerations about the short BUDs, it is also a good idea to question a long BUD from a pharmacy when others have indicated that their version of the product has a short BUD. There can be legitimate reasons for this variation such as a pharmacy having done an internal stability study versus a pharmacy using a USP default date. However, there may be other reasons for the longer date. It is known that drugs in aqueous liquid bases are more likely to degrade quickly compared to drugs in nonaqueous bases. While this is evident in USP's default BUDs, it is not a good idea to put all drugs in oil bases to extend the BUD. There are clinical considerations about whether it is appropriate to administer the drug with oil as well as considerations about if the drug characteristics like solubility allow for a high-quality formulation in oil and if it really is stable through the default BUD. If a pharmacy has a much longer BUD for a particular compound compared to others, research the drug as if you were going to compound it in-house. What is the longest BUD you could assign? If the pharmacy's BUD is longer, ask for the reference that supports the longer dating. If internal studies were used, determine if they were done with validated stability-indicating assay methods.

If you notice that the BUD for a particular drug, while sufficiently long, seems to vary with each prescription from a pharmacy, that may be an indication the pharmacy does anticipatory compounding of that particular product. Anticipatory compounding is a practice that allows pharmacies to make a larger batch of a compound that is frequently dispensed in anticipation of prescriptions that will be received in the coming weeks. An example of this is using a capsule machine to make a 300-count batch of gabapentin 50-mg capsules when only 30 are needed for the current prescription. A pharmacy may do this when they know they get several prescriptions for gabapentin 50-mg capsules a day and will quickly use the full 300 capsules. For anticipatory compounding, the BUD still starts on the date of compounding, so if one month the prescription is from a batch that was just made and the next month the prescription is filled with a batch that was made a couple weeks ago, the BUD will appear different. Generally, anticipatory compounding is only done for compounds that have BUDs significantly longer than the average duration prescribed.

Conclusion

Establishing an appropriate BUD is an essential part of compounding. There are a wide variety of factors that can affect drug stability, and the unique nature of each compound means that we often do not have all the information to know exactly how long a compounded formulation will remain stable before clinically significantly degradation occurs. Therefore, it is important to critically evaluate the information that is available and err on the conservative side when establishing a BUD.

References

1 (2022). CFR – Code of Federal Regulations title 21. https://www.accessdata.fda.gov/scripts/cdrh/cfdocs/cfcfr/CFRSearch.cfm?fr=225.1 (accessed 1 January 2023).
2 United States Pharmacopeial Convention (2022). USP general chapter <1151> pharmaceutical dosage forms. *USP Compounding Compendium*. Rockville, MD: USP.

3 (2022). CFR – Code of Federal Regulations title 21. https://www.accessdata.fda.gov/scripts/cdrh/cfdocs/cfcfr/CFRSearch.cfm?CFRPart=7 (accessed 22 September 2022).

4 United States Pharmacopeial Convention (2022). USP general chapter <1191> stability considerations in dispensing practice. *USP Compounding Compendium*. Rockville, MD: USP.

5 United States Pharmacopeial Convention (2022). USP general chapter <1149> guidelines for assessing and controlling the physical stability of chemical and biological pharmaceutical raw materials, intermediates, and dosage forms. *USP Compounding Compendium*. Rockville, MD: USP.

6 Trissel, L.A. (1983). Avoiding common flaws in stability and compatibility studies of injectable drugs. *Am. J. Hosp. Pharm.* 40 (7): 1159–1160.

7 Trissel, L.A. (1985). Evaluation of the literature on stability and compatibility of parenteral admixtures. *NITA* 8 (5): 365–369.

8 Trissel, L.A. and Flora, K.P. (1988). Stability studies: five years later. *Am. J. Hosp. Pharm.* 45 (7): 1569–1571.

9 Ray, G., Crook, M., West, N. et al. (1984). Comparison of the analysis of delta 9-tetrahydrocannabinol capsules by high-performance liquid chromatography and capillary gas chromatography. *J. Chromatogr.* 317: 455–462. https://doi.org/10.1016/s0021-9673(01)91685-1.

4

Identifying High-Quality Compounding Pharmacies

As discussed in Chapter 2, there is significant risk associated with the use of compounded products, but there is also a need to use them to appropriately treat patients in many cases. While it is true that some dosage forms present more risk than others, any dosage form can be compounded poorly or very well. The most significant predictor of the product quality is the quality of the compounding pharmacy preparing the compound. This concept also applies to veterinarians compounding for their own patients in that the better the adherence to quality standards, the better the end product quality will be. This chapter will focus on evaluating compounding pharmacy quality, and subsequent chapters will focus on preparing high-quality formulations in-house.

An easy method for evaluating the quality of compounding pharmacies is to ensure that they are legally compliant with state laws and applicable United States Pharmacopeia (USP) standards as the combination of these should produce compounds that meet a generally acceptable standard. However, a pharmacy simply saying they are compliant does not mean they actually are and there are a lot of potential areas that are not addressed in the regulations or USP standards that affect compounded product quality. Therefore, additional evaluation is needed. The following case examples will use historical website screenshots to show how a compounding pharmacy can say all the right things to look compliant on the surface but actually have several problems upon closer inspection.

Case Study 1

The New England Compounding Center (NECC) was a compounding pharmacy located in Framingham, MA. This pharmacy became a known name after becoming the center of the fungal meningitis outbreak that started in 2012. Additional details of the outbreak can be found in Chapter 1. This case study will look at how a pharmacy at the center of the largest public health crisis to ever result from a pharmaceutical drug had a booming business shipping sterile compounds throughout the United States [1].

Were there red flags about the quality of products from this pharmacy that should have served as a warning to prescribers? By 2012, the Internet had been used for marketing purposes for several years, so reviewing the website of NECC (neccrx.com) would have been the easiest way to get an initial look at the quality of the pharmacy. Today, we still commonly use a compounding pharmacy's website to decide if we want to prescribe drugs through them. Through archive.org, the following screenshots (see Figures 4.1–4.5) were obtained from the NECC website during 2011.

Drug Compounding for Veterinary Professionals, First Edition. Lauren R. Eichstadt Forsythe and Alexandria E. Gochenauer.
© 2023 John Wiley & Sons, Inc. Published 2023 by John Wiley & Sons, Inc.
Companion Website: www.wiley.com/go/forsythe/drug

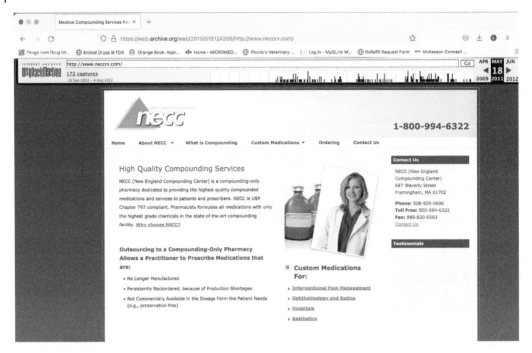

Figure 4.1 The homepage of the NECC website as it appeared on May 18, 2011. The webpage looks professional, contains contact information, and lists appropriate reasons why a compounded medication may be necessary. The welcome paragraph states that the pharmacy is "...dedicated to providing the highest quality compounded medications and services to patients and prescribers." There is also a link titled "Why choose NECC?"

These images show a professional webpage for a pharmacy that appears to value quality compounding and USP compliance. The information available talks about the cleanroom, the pharmacists' training in sterile compounding, and the quality control program. However, the final webpage image available is of the all-product recall that occurred in October 2012.

On December 13, 2018, a press release was issued detailing the conviction of an owner and four former NECC employees bringing the total convicted of federal charges to 11 former owners, executives, and employees. Those convicted include cleanroom pharmacists, verification pharmacists, the head pharmacist, and the former director of operations. The press release [1] includes the following quote from United States Attorney Andrew Lelling:

> These defendants were professionals who acted recklessly to the extreme detriment of public health. Over the course of years, the defendants callously disregarded patient health by cutting corners and prioritizing profits over safety. And they got away with it by defrauding federal and state regulators. The result was contaminated, deficient, deadly drugs that never should have been distributed.

According to the press release, the unsafe way several sterile products were prepared included "failure to properly sterilize NECC's drugs, failure to properly test NECC's drugs for sterility, and failure to wait for test results before sending the drugs to customers." These actions were in direct conflict with the quality standards described in the website screenshots. Other findings included the use of expired drug ingredients, NECC's lack of proper cleaning, and failure to act when environmental monitoring repeatedly detected mold and bacteria within the cleanrooms.

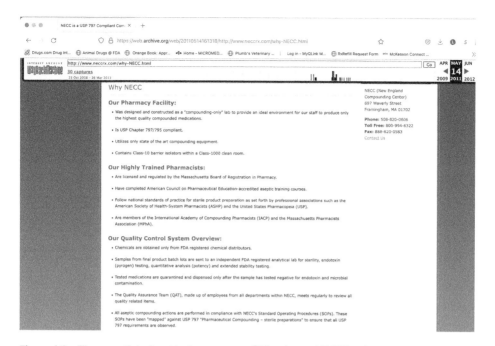

Figure 4.2 The page linked on the homepage as "Why choose NECC?" as it appeared on May 14, 2011. This page provides several details that would lead a visitor to believe this pharmacy prepares high-quality compounds. This page states that NECC facilities are USP 797/795 compliant and have Class-10 barrier isolators within a Class-1000 clean room. It also states that the pharmacists are licensed in MA, have completed American Council on Pharmaceutical Education (ACPE)-accredited aseptic training courses, follow American Society of Health-System Pharmacists (ASHP) and USP standards for sterile compounding, and are members of the International Academy of Compounding Pharmacists (IACP) and the Massachusetts Pharmacists Association (MPhA). This page also contains an overview of their quality control system. The quality control section states that samples from final product batches are sent to an FDA-registered analytical lab for sterility, endotoxin, potency, and stability testing and that these lots are quarantined and dispensed only after they have negative endotoxin and microbial contamination results from the submitted sample. According to this page, NECC also had a Quality Assurance Team that met to review all quality related items as well as SOPs designed to ensure all sterile compounding is done in accordance with USP 797.

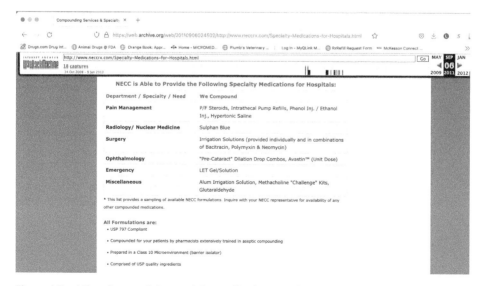

Figure 4.3 A list of some of the specialty medications provided for hospitals as of September 6, 2011. This page again states that the formulations are all prepared in compliance with USP 797, pharmacists are "extensively trained in aseptic compounding," and the medications are prepared in a Class 10 Microenvironment.

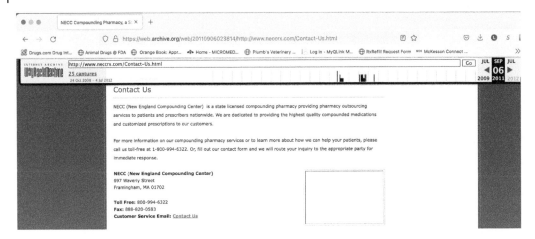

Figure 4.4 The Contact Us page of the NECC website as it appeared on September 6, 2011. This page again states that NECC is state-licensed and provides compounded medications nationwide. It also states, "We are dedicated to providing the highest quality compounded medications and customized prescriptions to our customers."

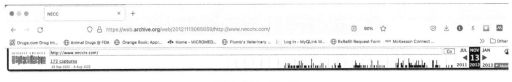

Figure 4.5 The NECC webpage detailing the nationwide recall of all products as it appeared on November 13, 2012.

Case Study 2

Franck's Pharmacy was a compounding pharmacy located in Ocala, FL known for sterile and nonsterile compounding for both veterinary and human patients. In 2009, a vitamin injection was compounded with 100 times more selenium than intended, which resulted in the deaths of 21 polo ponies competing in the US Open Polo Championship. In 2016, a $2.5M verdict was found against the pharmacy staff involved. The error first occurred in a mistake transcribing the prescription. When problems occurred in the compounding process due to the incorrect prescription transcription, the pharmacist overseeing the lab failed to verify the accuracy and appropriateness of the prescription they were attempting to prepare [2]. When looking at the Franck's Pharmacy website (francks.com) as it appeared prior to 2009, we are again met with promises of quality as shown in the screenshots (see Figures 4.6–4.8) obtained from archive.org.

Like with the NECC case, these webpage examples do not raise significant concern about using Franck's Pharmacy for a source of compounded products.

The remainder of this chapter will discuss what to evaluate and methods for evaluating compounding pharmacies to make an informed decision about pharmacies that can be counted on to provide high-quality products.

What to Evaluate

When evaluating a compounding pharmacy, it is important to consider general practices, staff skill level, familiarity with veterinary medicine, and the pharmacy culture. This section will describe each of these in more detail.

General Practices

This refers to the general pharmacy policies and procedures that are in place. Do they have them, do they reflect what is actually done, and do they comply with all relevant laws and best practices? Does the staff know where to locate policies and procedures? Is the pharmacy maintained in a clean and organized manner? Is there a feel that the staff is working like a well-oiled machine or is

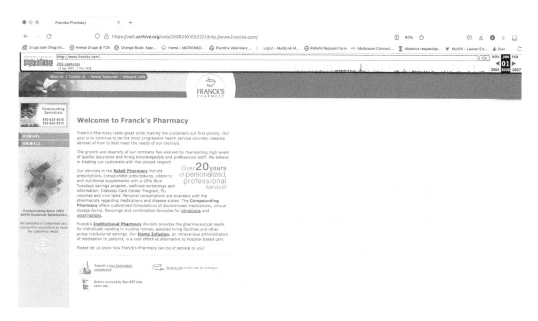

Figure 4.6   The homepage of the Franck's Pharmacy website as it appeared on January 1, 2006. The information appears standard.

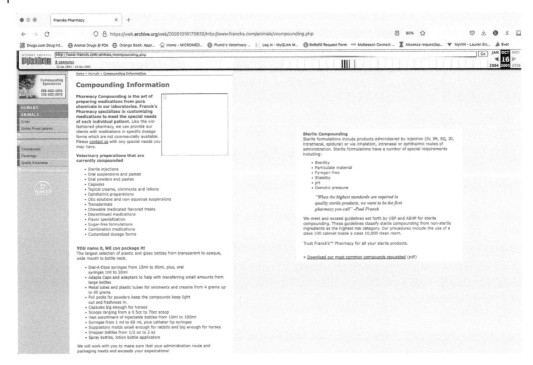

Figure 4.7 The Compounding Information webpage as it appeared on October 16, 2005. The information again is pretty standard. It does appear that the pharmacy prepares a large variety of products which could potentially increase the risk of errors or poor formulations. However, for a large pharmacy, that may not be unusual and is a risk that can be mitigated.

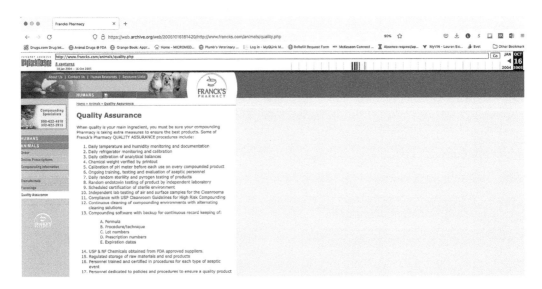

Figure 4.8 The Quality Assurance webpage for Franck's Pharmacy as it appeared on October 10, 2005. Again, there is nothing unusual and the USP boxes appear to all be checked.

it chaotic? Lack of clear policies and procedures can lead to a chaotic environment where there are varying levels of understanding of the appropriate process and expectations. Although there is often more than one acceptable way to do something, when everyone does the task differently, subsequent tasks are performed based on different expectations, which increases the risk of errors occurring. These general considerations are not specific to veterinary compounding but rather are the foundation that supports a high-quality compounding pharmacy of any type.

Staff Skill Level

Simply because someone is a pharmacist or a licensed pharmacy technician does not mean that they have extensive compounding experience. Compounding is a minor topic taught to varying degrees in pharmacy schools and pharmacy technician programs. In most cases, a highly skilled compounding pharmacist or technician got to that point through working in a compounding pharmacy and choosing to pursue additional education and training on the topic. Therefore, it is not practical to assume that only those already experienced in compounding will be hired. Instead, there should be a well-defined process in place for training new staff to ensure they are trained to handle the variety of formulations they will be tasked with preparing. Does the pharmacy have a training process and a competency check in place? Is there a process for periodically reevaluating the competency of their current staff? This is critical to ensuring that new staff are aware of all the nuances in the compounding process for various formulations as well as verifying continued competency of current staff.

Familiarity with Veterinary Medicine

Concepts pertaining to providing medications for animal patients are not core competencies in pharmacy school or pharmacy technician training programs. For someone to have knowledge of veterinary pharmacy, they need to have taken advantage of elective course work and/or pursued additional training or continuing education in that subject. While core compounding concepts are the same for both human and veterinary compounds, the formulations that are prepared, acceptable inactive ingredients, and other clinical considerations will be different. The best-quality compounds for animal patients are likely to come from compounding pharmacies with pharmacists (and ideally pharmacy technicians) that have at least a baseline knowledge of veterinary pharmacy concepts and how they differ from human pharmacy.

Pharmacy Culture

This is the vaguest of the concepts making it potentially difficult to evaluate. The culture of the compounding pharmacy should be such that they are a collaborative member of the care team where they are interested in engaging with clients and veterinarians to problem solve and determine possible options for difficult cases. These pharmacies will welcome requests for novel formulations but will critically evaluate the appropriateness prior to agreeing to prepare them. Veterinarians should feel confident that they can reach out to the pharmacist and suggest potential formulation ideas and that the pharmacist will provide insight on the appropriateness from their perspective including if the requested formulation is likely inappropriate. An example is with transdermal formulations. There are limited data on drugs that work transdermally. If a veterinarian requests a transdermal medication which the pharmacy does not currently prepare, the pharmacist should engage in a discussion of the likelihood of success as well as the potential risks associated with that drug/dosage form combination. Some medications are relatively low risk transdermally beyond the risk that it will not work as intended which the veterinarian may determine as a risk that they are willing to accept. However, a transdermal antibiotic intended to provide systemic blood levels carries a risk to both human and animal health beyond the current patient due to the low likelihood of successful therapy combined with a high likelihood of contributing to increased bacterial resistance. These are important discussions that do not occur in pharmacies that are willing to make anything a veterinarian will prescribe if a client is willing pay for it.

Ways to Evaluate Compounding Pharmacies

Both the case studies demonstrate why the evaluation of a compounding pharmacy beyond a website review is important to ensure that prescribed compounded medications are obtained from a high-quality pharmacy. The following sections describe methods in which to complete this evaluation.

Despite the cautions demonstrated in the case studies, reviewing a pharmacy's website is a quick and easy way to get initial information as long as it is not the sole source of evaluating the pharmacy. The following details can be obtained from the website.

- Pharmacy name: The full pharmacy name with correct spelling is helpful to use for verifying the pharmacy's licensure status and if there are any Food and Drug Administration (FDA) inspection reports or warning letters documented.
- Physical location: The physical location is an important piece of information to know as the pharmacy must be licensed in the state in which it is located. The pharmacy also needs to be licensed in any state that meds are shipped to.
- States the pharmacy will ship to: If you are not located in the same state that the pharmacy is in, it is important to verify that the pharmacy is able to ship to your state. Most pharmacies will include this information on their website; however, it is still important to verify that they have a license in good standing in your state. Which states a pharmacy will ship to is often a careful decision, and the reasons for not shipping to a certain state can vary. Each state will have different requirements for a pharmacy to obtain an out of state license. Requirements range from a license in good standing in the resident state to requiring a pharmacist be licensed in the state to requiring the pharmacy pay expenses for a board inspector to come do an in-person inspection of the pharmacy. The varying requirements result in additional state licensure being a strategic business decision for each pharmacy.
- 503b status: This information will likely be found on pharmacy websites that are 503b facilities, and it will appear as 503b or by referring to the pharmacy as an outsourcing facility. Typically, this status is something a pharmacy likes to promote, so it is often easily seen on the webpage. If there is no indication of 503a or 503b, then the pharmacy is likely 503a, but that fact can be verified by the methods discussed later in this chapter.
- Type of compounds prepared: A pharmacy may not list everything they prepare on their website. However, they should include information about the types of compounds they make. If you are looking for a sterile compound, it is important to verify that the pharmacy is equipped for sterile compounding. It can also be helpful to determine if the pharmacy specializes in the specific medications you will need or species you work with. For example, some pharmacies specialize in preparing equine medications. These pharmacies will likely be familiar with dosage forms commonly used in horses, and their staff likely has extensive experience preparing

these. That can be beneficial for something like an oral paste that may not be commonly prepared in some compounding pharmacies. Since oral pastes require a medication to be distributed evenly and then are filled into a dosing tube while maintaining even drug distribution and filling (i.e. no air pockets), this dosage form can take some practice to do well. Compounding pharmacists and technicians at an equine compounding pharmacy have likely been trained by people experienced in this dosage form.

– Contact information: This information should include how to reach a pharmacist with questions. The contact information is also necessary to ask some of the questions discussed below.

Looking Beyond the Pharmacy's Website

After getting some basic information from the pharmacy's website, the next step is to investigate licenses and certifications. Every 503a pharmacy needs to have a license in good standing with the state in which they are physically located. Some states require additional licensure based on type of compounding performed. For example, if a pharmacy prepares sterile compounds, and the state in which they are located requires a sterile compounding license, then the pharmacy needs to have the sterile compounding license. Licensure status can be determined through the state pharmacy board's website. Because different states include their pharmacy boards within different agencies, an easy way to find the pharmacy board's website for the state in question is to search for "_____ board of pharmacy" where the blank is the name of the state. For shipping out of state, the pharmacy is required to meet all licensure requirements in the state the medication is being shipped to. For example, if they want to ship sterile compounds to a state that requires a separate sterile compounding license, then they will need to have that additional sterile compounding license active and in good standing.

If the pharmacy is operating as a 503b outsourcing facility, they are required to be registered as an outsourcing facility with the FDA. This information can be found on the FDA page titled Registered Outsourcing Facilities which is where all outsourcing facilities are listed. You can also access FDA inspection forms (Form FDA-483) from this page for outsourcing facilities for which they have been issued. This FDA outsourcing facility list should be consulted to verify status of a pharmacy claiming to be a 503b facility and to determine the 503 status of a pharmacy that is not clear based on the website. In addition to FDA registration as an outsourcing facility, individual states often require a separate type of registration. In some states, 503b facilities may be registered as wholesalers and others may have an outsourcing designation. Like 503a pharmacies, 503b facilities must comply with the requirements of any state they are located in or shipping to in addition to federal requirements.

Form FDA-483 is an official list of observations made during an inspection that the investigator believes is a violation of the Food, Drug, and Cosmetic (FD&C) Act. The findings are listed in order of significance with the most severe being listed first. At the conclusion of the inspection, items on Form 483 are discussed with the establishment's senior management to ensure that everyone is clear on what is being communicated. Form 483 is not a final determination on FD&C Act violations, and management is encouraged to respond in writing with their corrective plan and to implement the plan as quickly as possible [3]. It is important to note that this form may be issued for any FDA inspection regardless of whether the pharmacy is a 503a or 503b facility.

Since 503b facilities are required to follow Current Good Manufacturing Practice and do have more uniform oversight of their compliance through the FDA, we can assume that products from these facilities are the most reliable. That said, it is still important to verify their licensure status and any items documented on a Form 483. For more information on 503b facilities and associated risks, refer to Chapter 2.

With 503a pharmacies, we see more variation of quality as USP requirements are often considered minimum best practices and allow for significant variation between pharmacies in how they are implemented. When looking at 503a pharmacies, one option is to look for Pharmacy Compounding Accreditation Board (PCAB) Accreditation. The PCAB is a voluntary compounding pharmacy accreditation that is completed through the Accreditation Commission for Healthcare (ACHC). The PCAB program was developed by eight US pharmacy organizations that saw the need to develop a voluntary program to give compounding pharmacies an opportunity to demonstrate their adherence to high-quality compounding practices. The PCAB designation also serves as an indicator to patients/clients that a compounding pharmacy has been independently evaluated and determined to comply with a high-quality standard [4]. This can be beneficial when it is become default to say that a compounding pharmacy is USP-compliant with little oversight of the accuracy of that statement. The devil is in the details, and many small USP details can fall through the cracks due to not being obvious sources of problems.

While seeing that a pharmacy has earned PCAB accreditation is an indicator of quality, the lack of accreditation does not necessarily indicate the opposite. A pharmacy may not be accredited because they do not meet the rigorous standards. However, they may also have decided the cost associated with the accreditation process would not result in significant benefit. A list of all the current PCAB accredited pharmacies can be found on the ACHC website under the "Find a Provider" section. This page provides the ability to search by state for accredited pharmacies and view details about each pharmacy's accreditation including the dates for which it is valid and if they have sterile and/or nonsterile accreditation [5]. Regardless of accreditation status, it is important to continue evaluating other aspects to gain a complete picture of the pharmacy.

In addition to the FDA Form 483 discussed above, it can also be beneficial to review warning letters and recalls associated with the pharmacy. There are two FDA webpages that are helpful for finding this information. The first is Compounding: Inspections, Recalls, and other Actions and covers pharmacies performing human drug compounding [6]. The second page is Inspections, Recalls, and Other Actions with Respect to Firms that Engage in Animal Drug Compounding [7]. If a pharmacy is involved in both human and veterinary compounding, they may appear on both lists with items pertaining to the relevant type of compounding listed. It is worthwhile to do a quick check of both lists to see if a pharmacy is listed on one or both. Items that may be found on these lists include issued Form 483s, which were discussed above, warning letters, information about recalls, and FDA press releases pertaining to the pharmacy. When evaluating these documents, it is important to consider the type of warning, recall or inspection finding, and the timeframe in which it occurred. For additional information on recalls, refer to Chapter 2. The following questions can be helpful when determining the applicability of the warnings.

1) How closely connected is the issue with the type of product I am looking to prescribe? For example, if the recalls and warnings all pertain to sterile compound sterility, that may not be particularly concerning if you are only looking to prescribe nonsterile compounds.
2) Are the documents recent (within the past few years) or older? If all documents are from more than five years prior, the problematic practices may have been effectively addressed.
3) Has pharmacy ownership, licensure status, and/or type of compounds prepared changed since the documents were issued? These changes may indicate a significant revamp of the pharmacy's quality standards that warrants consideration.

If a particular pharmacy you are interested in has items listed that are of unclear significance, tailor your questions for the pharmacist (discussed below) to find out a bit more about the problem.

After completing the online review described above, it is time to dig into more details which involve talking to people. Word of mouth is not likely to provide a lot of helpful information. Keep in mind that a colleague's experience likely represents only a very small percentage of the total compounds prepared by the pharmacy, so it may not be an indicator of total quality. However, do not discredit it completely. If a colleague has had issues with a compounding pharmacy, learn the details and keep that in mind as you further evaluate the pharmacy. At this point, consider how you want to go about getting additional insight. If you are local to the pharmacy, you could contact the pharmacy and request a meeting with the pharmacist in charge (PIC) and a tour of the facility. If you are not local, you can still request to speak with the PIC and schedule a time to do so.

What to Look for on a Tour

The following are some ideas of things to look for while touring a facility, but this list is not all-inclusive. If the facility is not willing to provide a tour or a tour is not feasible due to location, many of these items can be reframed into questions for the PIC.

1) Cleanliness of compounding spaces
2) Types of equipment used (e.g. do they have an ointment mill if they are preparing topical creams/ointments or transdermal products?)
3) Appropriate personal protective equipment for type of compounding performed
4) Policies and standard operating procedures (SOPs) relevant to the work being done
5) Defined cleanroom with restricted access if doing sterile compounding
6) A workflow that supports pharmacist oversight and verification
7) Master formulation records and thorough documentation of the quantities and details of the ingredients used for each compound
8) Quality checks throughout the compounding process for all formulation types

In addition to these points, keep in mind that you are looking for signs that quality may be decreased or corners are being cut. If you are unfamiliar with what baseline USP compliance looks like, this can be more difficult. However, if you can tour multiple compounding pharmacies with similar scopes, you will start to get a feel for what a standard level looks like.

Questions to Ask the Pharmacist in Charge

In an ideal scenario, you will have the opportunity to get a tour of the pharmacy and then meet with the PIC afterward to ask additional questions. However, if that is not feasible, you should still be able to contact the PIC and set up a time to talk with them in person or via phone or email. If you or a colleague have had a particular issue with a compound in the past, make sure to include a question or two that will find out what the pharmacy does to prevent that issue. If a pharmacy was listed on the FDA website with a Form 483, recall, warning, or press release, consider adding a question that will provide more information about what was done to address the issue(s). The following are questions to consider asking, but the list is not all-inclusive.

1) What veterinary and compounding training and experience has the pharmacy staff had?
   Rationale: Pharmacists and pharmacy technicians are trained on human pharmacy concepts. How to apply that information to veterinary patients is an elective topic. There are options for pharmacists and pharmacy technicians to learn more about veterinary pharmacy, but these are

not required components of training. Compounding is taught some in pharmacy training, but the amount of time spent on it is limited. Therefore, it is important to determine that the pharmacists (and ideally the technicians) have experience and/or training in both the veterinary and compounding components.

2) How long have they been making a particular formulation? (Tailor this question to the specific formulations you are interested in such as sterile products.)

Rationale: If you are looking to find a compounding pharmacy for ophthalmic compounds, a pharmacy that has been preparing ophthalmic preparations for many years without documented problems may earn more prescriber confidence than a pharmacy that has just started preparing ophthalmic products. While compounding has a lot of regulations and best practices, it is still a bit of an art form. More experience with a dosage form often means higher quality. If the pharmacy is new to preparing a dosage form, ask what was done to ensure they have strong policies, procedures, and training in place. Newness to something may represent a risk, but that risk can be mitigated with conscious effort.

3) How do they develop new formulations?

Rationale: A creative compounding pharmacist can make just about anything, but that does not mean it should be made. There are a variety of considerations that go into whether a compound should be made. For a complete list, see Chapter 2. When creating new formulations there needs to be a process in place where a pharmacist is reviewing the appropriateness from both a formulation and a clinical appropriateness perspective. A pharmacy that is willing to make anything requested by a veterinarian is a red flag as the pharmacist should be doing research and engaging in additional discussion prior to agreeing to make a new formulation.

4) How do they determine the beyond-use dates for their products?

Rationale: Beyond-use dates may be determined by utilizing the default dating that is provided by USP in chapters 795 and 797. However, longer beyond-use dates may also be used if there are stability studies to support them. See Chapter 3 for a full discussion on what is and is not acceptable when determining beyond-use dates.

5) What quality testing is done?

Rationale: USP chapters outline the minimum quality checks that should occur. However, additional testing on a batch or intermittent basis can be useful to identify process or training problems that need corrected. At a minimum, the pharmacy should meet USP requirements, and a pharmacy that does additional quality testing may be desirable. The pharmacy should also have a plan in place to address any out of specification results that are found.

6) At what points in the compounding process do quality checks occur?

Rationale: There should be multiple stop points in the preparation of a compound where a second person is verifying the accuracy of the steps completed so far. Common check points are when ingredients have been pulled, when they have been weighed/measured, and when the formulation is complete. However, pharmacies may utilize different check points based on the risk analysis of their compounding process. There should be sufficient checks in place to prevent human error from making it through the entire compounding process.

7) How are reported adverse effects documented and addressed?

Rationale: Compounding pharmacies need to have a method for documenting adverse effects and product problems that are reported to them. They also need a process in place for determining if there is sufficient evidence that a recall is necessary for the product lot. A high-quality compounding pharmacy should have a plan in place before they need it.

8) What is the training and supervision process for new staff?

Rationale: The defined checkpoints described above are designed to catch human error such as incorrect ingredient selection or a math error. However, it will not necessarily identify problems due to lack of training such as poor compounding techniques. It is important that a comprehensive training process is in place to determine when someone has proven the skillset to prepare compounds without someone standing over their shoulder the entire time.

In addition to the questions above, there are two additional questions I like to ask regarding formulation development. These can certainly be asked to the PIC, but it might be more telling of the general culture to ask these questions of another pharmacist or compounding technician. If I have a limited window talking to someone and am only going to ask two questions, these are the ones I ask. I use one question to determine the pharmacy's compliance with legal requirements such as not duplicating commercial products, and I use the second question to evaluate if formulation requests are being critically evaluated. The correct answer to both of the following questions should be "no."

1) This first question I ask is whether they will compound _____ (insert example of expensive and readily available commercial product).
   Rationale: It is not legal to compound a duplicate of a commercial product unless that product is on backorder. If the response is that they cannot compound an identical strength but will compound a very similar strength (e.g. 95 mg instead of 100 mg), then that is unlikely to be a clinically significant difference thus raising concern that they are aware of the legality of compounding a duplicate and have intentionally identified a way to circumvent the law.
2) The second question I ask is whether they will compound transdermal enrofloxacin.
   Rationale: While this may be legal, transdermal antibiotics are much more likely to result in bacterial resistance than efficacy, enrofloxacin is a fluoroquinolone that is a class of high-priority antibiotics for humans making resistance more concerning, and there is a published study showing that enrofloxacin is not absorbed transdermally [8]. All these points make this a bad public health decision due to concerns surrounding antibiotic resistance.

Conclusion

Mindful prescribing of compounded medications requires addressing the risk: benefit ratio of using a compound, and an important risk to consider is the quality of the compounded product. While some dosage forms carry more risk than others, any dosage form can be made very well or very poorly, and the quality of the compounding pharmacy is a strong predictor of the quality that can be expected. It is a responsibility of the prescribing veterinarian to understand what makes a compounding pharmacy a reliable choice for compounded medications. Owing to the time requirement to evaluate the quality of a compounding pharmacy, the authors recommend finding a couple local compounding pharmacies and a couple national compounding pharmacies that can be recommended to clients with confidence.

References

1 (2018). December 13, 2018: owner and four former employees of New England Compounding Center convicted following trial. FDA. https://www.fda.gov/inspections-compliance-enforcement-and-criminal-investigations/press-releases/december-13-2018-owner-and-four-former-employees-new-england-compounding-center-convicted-following (accessed 7 October 2022).

2 Crisco, A. (2016). $2.5M verdict slaps compounding lab and pharmacist in trial over poisoning deaths of 21 polo ponies. https://blog.cvn.com/2.5m-verdict-slaps-compounding-lab-and-pharmacist-in-trial-over-poisoning-deaths-of-21-polo-ponies (accessed 7 October 2022).

3 (2020). FDA Form 483 frequently asked questions. FDA. https://www.fda.gov/inspections-compliance-enforcement-and-criminal-investigations/inspection-references/fda-form-483-frequently-asked-questions (accessed 7 October 2022).

4 Accreditation for compounding pharmacies. NCPA. https://ncpa.org/accreditation-for-compounding-pharmacies (accessed 7 October 2022).

5 Compounding pharmacy – ACHC. https://www.achc.org/compounding-pharmacy (accessed 7 October 2022).

6 (2022). Compounding: inspections, recalls, and other actions. FDA. https://www.fda.gov/drugs/human-drug-compounding/compounding-inspections-recalls-and-other-actions (accessed 7 October 2022).

7 (2022). Inspections, recalls, and other actions with respect to firms that engage in animal drug compounding. FDA. https://www.fda.gov/animal-veterinary/animal-drug-compounding/inspections-recalls-and-other-actions-respect-firms-engage-animal-drug-compounding (accessed 7 October 2022).

8 Karriker, M., Wiebe, V., Parsons, K., and Stanley, S. (2005). Plasma concentrations of enrofloxacin in cats after transdermal administration of a PLO gel formulation. ACVIM.

5

Formulation Development

Dosage Forms

Active pharmaceutical ingredients (APIs) mixed with inactive ingredients or "excipients" are formulated into a variety of dosage forms. Compounded medications are available in commonly used dosage forms such as capsules and oral suspensions as well as less familiar dosage forms like transdermal gels or intranasal solutions. Oral dosage forms, such as the capsules in Figure 5.1 below, are the most common mechanism of drug delivery and provide the advantage of predetermined doses and portability.

Oral Administration

Liquid compounded medications are beneficial for medicating many animal species. Cats can be difficult to pill, and following the administration of certain caustic drugs (e.g. doxycycline), there is a risk of gastrointestinal erosion due to their horizontal orientation [2]. Exotic pets, particularly birds and guinea pigs, also require liquid medications on account of their size and a common goal of clinicians to treat patients appropriately while causing the least amount of stress. Prescribing a liquid medication can also be a safer option to ensure that an accurate dose is given every time. Commonly prepared oral liquid dosage forms include solutions, suspensions, and syrups.

Oral Solutions

An oral solution is a mixture where one substance is fully dissolved into another. The oral solution will be clear, or free of visible particulates, and at no point in time should the ingredients separate or settle to the bottom of the bottle. If separation does occur, this is a sign of a stability problem. A substance dissolves well when it has a small particle size and appropriate solubility for the vehicle. If there are particles visible on the bottle or in the syringe when drawing up the dose, a solution has not been effectively prepared as there is either drug or excipient that is not dissolved. Solutions are advantageous as a dosage form as phase separation will not occur like it can with suspensions and emulsions. Solutions also do not require disintegration and dissolution, meaning that they will be absorbed faster. Bitter taste is also more easily masked with oral solutions. A disadvantage of solutions is that they are less stable than other dosage forms, and degradation may occur even if appropriate excipients, such as antioxidants, buffers, and preservatives, are added. If drug solubility is not exceeded in a formulation, this dosage form is extremely easy to compound.

Drug Compounding for Veterinary Professionals, First Edition. Lauren R. Eichstadt Forsythe and Alexandria E. Gochenauer.
© 2023 John Wiley & Sons, Inc. Published 2023 by John Wiley & Sons, Inc.
Companion Website: www.wiley.com/go/forsythe/drug

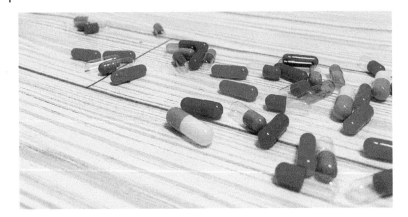

Figure 5.1 Colored gelatin capsules.

Oral Suspensions

An oral suspension is a mixture where one substance is suspended in another substance. An oral suspension requires the product to be shaken well prior to each use, whereas a solution does not. If the substance does not redisperse upon shaking or cakes at the bottom of the bottle, that may be a sign of instability and/or problems with the formulation. When developing a formulation, it is important that the formulation is thick enough to keep the drug particles suspended for a long enough period of time to accurately measure out a dose without the formulation being so thick that it is difficult to shake, and there are concerns about proper drug dispersion. The oral suspension will appear more opaque or cloudy due to the ingredient particles floating throughout it. It should be noted, however, that suspensions can "break," and the formation of crystals should not be mistaken for suspended drug particles. In the case that crystals form or drug powder clumps together and cannot be redispersed, the preparation should be thrown out and remade. Advantages of oral suspensions are that drugs that have poor solubility and cannot be administered in solution can be utilized, and they have a higher rate of bioavailability than capsules and tablets. Disadvantages are that they are not as bioavailable as solutions, and dosing accuracy is not as reliable since it depends on if the mixture is appropriately shaken, and the drug redispersed prior to each dose administered. Oral suspensions are easy to compound as long as the active drug is ground into a fine powder allowing for proper incorporation into the vehicle.

Oral Syrups

An oral syrup is a mixture where one substance is dissolved into another substance that is thick, sweet, and sticky. Simple syrup is a clear vehicle that is commonly used for compounded oral syrups, but there are also flavored syrups (e.g. grape and cherry) available. By definition, syrups primarily consist of a solution of sugar in water. The inherent sweetness present in this vehicle makes it an excellent option for reducing the perceived bitterness of medications. Perceived sweet and bitter tastes have an antagonistic relationship in that they mutually suppress each other. The preference for sweet versus bitter flavoring is innate, but in general sweet is preferred among the majority of species due to bitter taste evolutionarily indicating the presence of toxins. One advantage of oral syrups is that similar to oral solutions, they are monophasic, signifying that no phase separation can occur. They also have a relatively high stability and are palatable in taste. Disadvantages of syrups are their potential for bacterial growth and unsuitability for drugs that are not water soluble due to their aqueous nature. Oral syrups are easy to compound but, due to their sugar-based vehicle, tend to be stickier and messier than other oral liquid preparations.

Medicating animal patients poses a variety of problems, which have the potential to be addressed through innovative solutions. This problem gives the compounder the option to prepare a new dosage form – oral treats. Solid compounded medications are beneficial in instances where there are few manufactured strengths available, especially for drugs with a narrow therapeutic index. They also provide the necessary treatment while avoiding allergies to ingredients such as preservatives, dyes, and other excipients. In addition, solid dosage forms are less likely to degrade giving them longer beyond-use dates (BUDs) than other dosage forms. Commonly compounded solid oral dosage forms include capsules, tablets, and treats.

Oral Capsules

Oral capsules are a dosage form in which medication in powder form, along with powdered excipient (e.g. filler), is encapsulated inside gelatin. Oral capsules are easier to customize with regard to strength or lack of ingredients than oral tablets. They also offer the option of opening the capsule and using the powder inside mixed with food, water, or another substance if recommended by the veterinarian. In some instances, multiple drugs can also be incorporated into the same capsule to decrease the number of separate medications that need to be administered, but caution is warranted due to the potential for the drugs to interact with each other and affect the stability of one or both.

Combining two different medications in the same capsule is an option when the patient is taking medications that will not require a dosage adjustment, that the patient will be taking long term, and that have low-density active ingredients or smaller strengths, which allows them to fit into an appropriate size capsule together. Combining two medications is not an option when the medication(s) has a narrow therapeutic index, drug interactions exist, or the medication requires tapering or adjustment based on laboratory values throughout the course of therapy. The compounder should be cautious about combining two medications together, especially when the patient has not taken both of them previously, as serious side effects from one or both of the medications can occur or there may be a drug interaction that has not been previously documented that can render one or both of the medications inactive. While a more pharmaceutically elegant product is produced by compounding the medications into a capsule, a similar effect can be obtained by the client placing manufactured or compounded tablets into an empty gelatin capsule prior to administration. This works best when the medications are tablets that are small or small fractions that will easily fit into an appropriately sized capsule. A common example is placing a quarter of a clopidogrel tablet along with any other medications given at that time into an empty gelatin capsule to decrease the number of separate medications as well as mask the bitterness that is exposed when clopidogrel is quartered.

Oral capsules can be compounded by hand-packing them each individually or by utilizing a capsule machine. Both hand-packing and capsule machines require packing statistics prior to preparing a formulation to confirm the amount of API and excipients to combine and are a bit of an art form to prepare consistently. Packing statistics also need to be completed any time a new product or lot number is received to guarantee consistency and strength within $\pm 10\%$. One exception to completing packing statistics is with manufactured capsules that contain beads (e.g. itraconazole, omeprazole, and tamsulosin). The beads can be weighed out into even quantities to allow for the preparation of smaller strength capsules. An example of this is weighing the full contents of a tamsulosin 0.4-mg capsule and dividing the contents equally into four empty capsules to create tamsulosin 0.1-mg capsules.

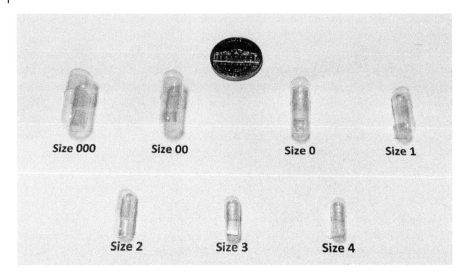

Figure 5.2 Oral capsule sizes.

There are many advantages to compounded capsules as they are the most versatile of all the compounded dosage forms. There is a myriad of colored capsules available, which can allow the compounder to color-code their formulations. Also, there is a range of sizes (000, 00, 0, 1, 2, 3, and 4), as seen in Figure 5.2, that make it easy to administer medication to a variety of species. Disadvantages to this dosage form include the requirement of a capsule machine for preparing large quantities, the calculations that must be completed to ensure that the compounded medication is prepared in the correct strength, the techniques that must be mastered to ensure consistently filled capsules, and the time that it takes to prepare a batch of capsules. Hand-packing and splitting beads are both relatively easy compounding procedures. The use of a capsule machine introduces additional equipment and requires knowledge for use, making it slightly more difficult to prepare large amounts of capsules than hand-packing. The compounder should also be aware that purchasing a capsule machine has strict requirements including providing the practitioners DEA number.

Oral Tablets
Oral tablets are a dosage form in which medication in powder form and powdered excipient (e.g. binders and lubricants) have been compressed together. For dosage adjustments, oral tablets can be easily scored. Molded tablet machines are used in the preparation of tablets. Oral tablets have natural small fissures throughout, so they will break down when exposed to water, with orally disintegrating tablet formulations dissolving far more rapidly than others. It can be advantageous to compound tablets due to their physical and chemical stability; however, it can also be disadvantageous because they absorb more slowly in the gastrointestinal tract (GI) tract than oral liquids due to the need for disintegration. Compounded tablets are also not a feasible dosage form for highly unpalatable or irritating medications. The process of compounding tablets is more difficult than capsules as the dosage form must withstand mechanical damage without falling apart and maintain its stability under a variety of conditions. Compressed tablets, those that are formed by compressing the ingredients using a steel punch, contain a slew of excipients to allow for their stability, both physically and chemically, which also contributes to

the difficulty level of preparing the formulation. Therefore, the preparation of compounded tablets is typically limited to large compounding pharmacies.

Oral Treats

Oral treats are a dosage form in which medication in powder form, along with excipient, is molded into the requested shape and packaged for freshness. Oral treats are formulated like regular pet treats and are a great option for pets that are difficult to administer oral tablets, capsules, or liquids to. Premade "base" is available from several compounding companies that is extremely easy to use. For patients that have diet restrictions or are picky eaters, crushed hard treats can also be used in combination with gelatin to make a treat base. Treats can be made in basic round molds, and bone- and fish-shaped molds are also offered to provide the look of a standard treat. The only shape requirement is that the mold be calibrated to create uniform weight treats. Oral treats as a dosage form are advantageous as food-motivated dogs and cats will readily accept it, and it is less stressful to administer than other oral solids or liquids. A disadvantage to this dosage form is that an additional piece of equipment, a hot plate, is needed to properly melt the gelatin or base. If the mold is not properly "greased," the treats may also get stuck and break apart upon removal. Compounding oral treats is relatively easy once the compounder has developed their step-by-step process for preparation, but a good technique must be used to ensure consistently prepared treats for accurate dosing.

Other oral dosage forms include emulsions, pastes, and powders. There are few monographs available for these oral dosage forms; however, they provide valuable forms of administration for some drugs and species.

Oral Emulsions

Oral emulsions are a dosage form that contains at least two immiscible liquids, such as oil and water, where one of the liquids is dispersed throughout the other in the form of small droplets. This is accomplished with the addition of an emulsifying agent. When oil is dispersed as small droplets throughout a continuous water phase, it is termed an oil-in-water (o/w) emulsion. When water is dispersed as small droplets throughout a continuous oil phase, it is termed a water-in-oil (w/o) emulsion. These are thermodynamically unstable systems with the w/o emulsion having less stability [3]. The stability of an emulsion can be easily determined by looking at the size of the globules present. Emulsions that are stable will have smaller globules. An example of a temporary emulsion – due to the lack of an emulsifier – is the combination of olive oil and balsamic. If the two are mixed all at once or in equal amounts, they will not combine appropriately. However, if the olive oil is slowly added to the balsamic while quickly mixing, then droplets will disperse throughout and create a nicely blended vinaigrette. Examples of commercial drugs that are emulsions include Diprivan (propofol), Baytril Otic (silver sulfadiazine and enrofloxacin), and over-the-counter oral mineral oil emulsions. The use of emulsions is advantageous for drugs that are hydrophilic and lipophilic as well as drugs that are unpalatable. Oral emulsions are less stable than oral solids and oral liquids as they can experience the following phenomena.

– Flocculation: Colloidal particles come out of suspension and form sediment.
– Creaming: Dispersed particles migrate to the surface of the emulsion.
– Coalescence: Smaller drops/globules combine to form larger drops/globules (irreversible).
– Breaking: Separation of the oil and water phases into two components.

Emulsions can be very complex systems that are thermodynamically unstable without the presence of an emulsifier. They are much more difficult to prepare correctly than other compounded formulations.

Oral Pastes

Oral pastes are semisolid dosage forms in which medication in powder form is distributed throughout an appropriate vehicle. Oral pastes are commonly used for administering medications to horses as they are convenient and forgo requiring the horse to accept the medication mixed in their food. The viscosity of the paste may affect the client's ability to administer it appropriately. If this occurs, they can modify the tip of the syringe by cutting it with a pair of scissors. When compounding oral pastes, filling the dosing syringe requires a skilled compounder to ensure that the thick paste is uniformly packed without air pockets that would affect the dosing accuracy. Pastes allow for a larger particle size of drug than suspensions making them beneficial for large doses of medications. One disadvantage of this dosage form is that phase separation may occur, and it would not be visually apparent until administration and, even then, may be missed resulting in inaccurate dosing. Compounding this dosage form is similar in difficulty to oral suspensions as long as the drug has already been proven to incorporate well into the vehicle as with formulas in the Compounding Compendium.

Oral Powders

Powders are a dosage form that is a dry, solid substance comprised of one or more finely ground drugs. This dosage form can contain excipients but does not have to and can be designed for topical application or oral ingestion. This dosage form has been around the longest due to the ease of preparation and administration. Powders can be utilized topically in a variety of areas including wounds in and around the mouth and the throat, and it can be an effective method for administering oral medications mixed with food. For topical administration, to provide complete coverage of the area (mouth or throat), powders can be applied using an insufflator. An insufflator is a device that has a bulbous end that collapses in on itself and directs powder through a long nozzle. Oral powders can also be incorporated into food or given alone. For horses, oral powders are often combined with lactose and a flavor, such as green apple or molasses, and dosed by the scoop.

Careful calculations are required to ensure that the amount of drug per scoop is defined. Understanding the science of mixing is important when preparing powders as they must be mixed effectively. Effective mixing occurs when geometric dilution, further discussed in Chapter 6, is used. To ensure that powders can be mixed appropriately, they are triturated, spatulated, sifted, or tumbled. Trituration is the process of grinding powder using a mortar and pestle. Spatulation is when powders are mixed on a pill tile/ointment slab or in a mortar using a powder spatula. Spatulation can only be utilized with powders that have the same densities. Sifting is a process that is beneficial when there are large particles intact after trituration. The powder is run through a sieve, which allows for the removal of any larger clumps. Finally, tumbling is a method for mixing powders where they are introduced into the same container which is then shaken or rotated. This method is utilized for powders with different densities. An electric mortar and pestle (EMP) or unguator EMP can perform this as an automated process and be set to the correct speed and sufficient mixing time. These pieces of equipment are very expensive and are not as commonly used in 503a pharmacies. Powders have the advantage of not requiring disintegration in the GI tract and are more stable than oral liquid dosage forms but are more likely to be denied by veterinary patients due to palatability issues. Compounding this formulation by hand is relatively easy, and appropriate mixing times can be determined using a colored tracer.

Transdermal Administration

Transdermal compounded medications are designed for medication delivery through the skin and into the bloodstream, providing a systemic effect. Transdermal compounded medications are easy to apply and bypass the need for oral medications that may be difficult to administer. This dosage form can be advantageous as it avoids hepatic first pass metabolism for drugs that have poor oral bioavailability [4]. Transdermal medications can be compounded into gels, ointments, or creams depending on the needs of the patient and the properties of the drug. Gels have been commonly used for transdermal drug delivery as they are easily absorbed, noncomedogenic, and can be used in intertriginous areas [5]. Ointments contain less than 20% water making them a poor choice for moisture bearing areas; however, they are beneficial when a high degree of occlusion is needed [5]. Creams have the most benefit when used on areas where there is little to no hair and when no occlusive effect is required [5]. Transdermal medications should be compounded utilizing the API as the source of drug instead of modifying a commercially available dosage form as this creates a higher quality product by eliminating the absorption effects of excipients from commercial products.

While administering drugs across the skin is an appealing option for administration in difficult patients, the unpredictability with which drugs are absorbed transdermally limits the usefulness of this dosage form. There are limited data on drugs that can be used for transdermal application, but it is known that not every medication should be compounded into a transdermal form. Transdermal delivery is more effective with the drug characteristics of low molecular weight (<500 Da) and moderate lipophilicity [6]. Drugs with narrow therapeutic indices should never be compounded into a transdermal product due to the likelihood that the drug will either be subtherapeutic or toxic because of unpredictable absorption. Other factors that affect absorption include the skin characteristics of the species and site of application as well as the presence of any of the wide variety of chemicals that act as penetration modifiers. This dosage form is easy to compound, but this ease often leads to inappropriate use, so caution in prescribing and compounding is advised. Therefore, it is recommended to limit the use of transdermal compounds to those drugs with studies showing efficacy by this route and utilize the studied formulations.

Topical Administration

Topical compounded medications act locally using a vehicle that carries the drug allowing it to be absorbed into the skin. They are differentiated from transdermal medications by the level of skin penetration. Topical medications do not reach below the epidermis limiting them to local effects, while transdermal medications penetrate the epidermis and dermis leading to system effects. Topical administration is beneficial as it can prevent systemic side effects of oral medications and provide an alternative for patients that cannot be pilled. Ease of administration of topical compounded medications is aided by the variety of dosage forms, which include solutions, ointments, shampoos, mousses, creams, gels, and emulsions. Transdermal compounded medications, as discussed in the previous paragraph, provide effective topical delivery and can be categorized under gels, creams, or ointments depending on the vehicle utilized. It is important to remember that, depending on the location of administration, topical administration may result in oral ingestion through grooming if the patient is not monitored. Therefore, care should be taken to ensure that the client is provided with details on how to prevent this, especially if the topical formulation has the potential to be orally toxic.

Topical Solutions
Topical solutions have the same properties as described above for oral solutions with the exception that ingredients used may not be safe for oral administration. The active ingredient may be dissolved in a variety of vehicles such as water, ethoxy diglycol, or alcohol. These formulations are commonly used for the administration of eye drops, ear drops, or to an area of inflammation. A topical solution may be dispensed in an oral dispensing bottle for ease of use, and

therefore, it should be denoted on the prescription label or using auxiliary labels that the medication is not for oral use. Topical solutions can also be dispensed in a spray bottle to improve the ease of administration. Topical solutions are extremely easy to compound and convenient for the client to use. A disadvantage of this formulation is that it does not last on the skin for an extended period of time and may be groomed off by the patient. The compounder must also take drug solubility into account when selecting a base.

Topical Ointments

Topical ointments are a dosage form in which the active ingredient is mixed into a thick, oily base. This preparation absorbs into the skin very slowly but can enhance the penetration of the active ingredient due to its occlusive properties. The oil-based vehicle will leave a film behind that is protective and ideal for dry skin. This formulation is advantageous as the active ingredient has a longer contact time with the affected site, while a disadvantage is that it can be groomed off by the patient and may stain clothes and furniture. Topical ointments are relatively easy to compound with the correct equipment – an ointment slab and spatula.

Topical Shampoos

Topical shampoos contain a solution or suspension composed of an anionic surfactant [7]. This preparation is intended to be applied to the hair/fur, being used as a vehicle for dermatologic agents, and then rinsed off after a predetermined time period. Compounded topical shampoos provide the ability to control the amount of every ingredient in them, preventing patients from being exposed to high concentrations of medications that are not safe for them. The client can partially control the contact time by allowing the shampoo to remain on the affected area prior to washing off. As shampoos can be washed off, there is a significant decrease in the chance of the medication being ingested. The disadvantage of topical shampoos is that they often require the client to bathe their animal two to three times per week in order to see an effect.

Topical Mousses

Topical mousses are dosage forms that contain an effective amount of API, an occlusive agent, an aqueous solvent, and an organic cosolvent [8]. The API must be insoluble in both water and the occlusive agent in order to produce the foam composition. The dosage form is a light and airy texture that enhances the dispersibility of the product. When a topical shampoo is not a feasible option, a topical mousse may be utilized in its place as it does not need to be washed off. This preparation combines a variety of active ingredients with inactive ingredients that soothe the area. Topical compounded mousses are ideal for larger areas of the body and areas with hair as they are absorbed quickly into the skin. A disadvantage to a topical mousse formulation is that the product stays on the animal and can be groomed off, leading to systemic concerns, or transfer to another member of the household.

Topical Emulsions

Emulsified systems are used for a variety of topical products. Emulsified lotions will have a lower viscosity than creams and ointments, but all are popular for external use. With topical emulsions, the compounder can select a suitable vehicle (cream, gel) for the compound's intended use, which provides control of the product's appearance, degree of oiliness, and viscosity. W/o emulsions are commonly used for dry skin as they have a thicker viscosity and increased degree of oiliness. A disadvantage to a topical emulsion formulation is that it may be difficult to prepare with an increased chance of breaking compared to other topical formulations.

Topical Creams

Topical creams are a dosage form in which the active ingredient is mixed into a vehicle that is a water base. Topical creams are semisolid emulsions that can be easily spread onto the skin and are beneficial for conditions that have large treatment areas. The water-based vehicle allows for the drug to be absorbed quickly into the skin without leaving behind residue. Topical creams are easier to prepare than other emulsions as they are o/w as opposed to w/o; however, they still have a higher potential to break than other topical formulations.

Topical Gels

Topical gels are a dosage form in which the active ingredient is mixed into a vehicle that is a water or combination water and alcohol base. This preparation turns into a liquid rapidly when it comes into contact with the skin and is beneficial for areas with large amounts of hair as it will disperse well. If a combination water and alcohol base is used, then it can be drying to the skin. Topical gels generally leave a thin residue on the skin after they dry. This formulation can be advantageous as it dries quicker than other topical formulations. One disadvantage is that some drugs may require the combination base of water and alcohol, which is less beneficial at affected sites that are inflamed.

Otic Administration

Otic compounded medications are applied to the outer ear or into the auditory canal to treat an ear infection. They are a great preparation for animals that have resistant or recurrent infections or have concomitant conditions that preclude the use of a specific ingredient such as a steroid. Otic formulations can be customized based on cytology and culture results, which helps prevent the formation of antibiotic resistance, and local administration results in higher drug concentrations at the site of infection. The dosage form utilized is often dependent on the patient's therapeutic needs and which drugs are being utilized. Typically, otic compounded medications include some combination of antibacterial, antifungal, and anti-inflammatory drugs.

Otic Solutions

An otic solution is the easiest and most commonly prepared otic compound. Like oral and topical solutions, it will be clear and at no point in time will the ingredients separate or settle. Otic solutions are extremely easy to compound, customize, and administer to patients. One disadvantage of this formulation is that the contact time may not be long enough as veterinary patients have a tendency to shake their heads following the installation of ear drops, leading to the solution being forced out of the ear. Also, administration in general can be poor as the drops intended for the ear may not reach the ear canal.

Otic Suspensions

An otic suspension is a mixture where one substance is suspended in another substance. An otic suspension requires the product to be shaken well prior to each use, whereas a solution does not. Often this preparation will contain both lipid soluble and aqueous components. If the substance does not redisperse upon shaking or cakes at the bottom of the bottle, that is an indication of a problem with the formulation. The preparation of an otic suspension should utilize the micronized version of the active ingredient to allow for proper absorption in the outer ear. Poloxamer gels can also be a useful vehicle for otic medications and are being included under this section as the active ingredient is dispersed throughout the gel. Poloxamer gels allow for increased contact time in the ear as they have a thin, water-like viscosity at cooler temperatures and become thick and gel like at higher temperatures. This leads to the preparation coating the area for an extended period of time. Formulations utilizing poloxamer gels are often referred to as "otic packs" due to them "packing the ear" with medication. Otic suspensions are relatively easy to compound, but those made with poloxamer gels require an understanding of the vehicle. The main disadvantages of otic suspensions are that the client must shake the medication sufficiently for the correct amount of drug to be instilled, and like otic solutions, otic suspensions can easily be "forced" out of the ear via head shaking.

Otic Ointments

Otic ointments are a dosage form in which the API is mixed into a thick, oily base. This preparation absorbs into the skin in the ear very slowly but can enhance the penetration of the active ingredient due to its occlusive properties. The oil-based vehicle will leave a film behind that is protective. Otic ointments are not frequently used but can be applied directly to the exterior portions of the ear. This otic formulation is advantageous as it stays on the affected site much better than solutions or suspensions, while a disadvantage is its occlusive properties as moisture within the ear has likely contributed to the current otic problem.

Other Routes of Administration

Rectal Solutions

Rectal solutions are a mixture where one substance is fully dissolved into another. This preparation is intended to be used like an enema or irrigation. Rectal solutions are beneficial in that they have faster absorption rates when compared to solid dosage forms that require disintegration or dissolution in order to release the drug [9]. Drugs that are more lipophilic or vehicles that contain fatty bases may be a rate-limiting step for drug absorption, whereas hydrophilic bases will produce a more sustained release effect [9]. Aqueous vehicles are available that improve the contact time of the preparation with the site of application, enhancing solubility in the rectal fluid. However, the solution needs to then be lipophilic enough to cross into the epithelium. An optimal balance between hydrophilicity and lipophilicity is key for the effective delivery of rectal solutions. In humans, rectal suppositories are commonly compounded, but this dosage form has less utility in veterinary patients due to the tendency to expel the suppository before it can dissolve and release the medication.

Intranasal Solutions

Intranasal solutions are also a mixture where one or more substances are fully dissolved into another. This preparation is intended to be used like nasal irrigation but with the benefit of medicating the area or rapidly delivering medication. Solutions that are applied nasally provide relief that is the most efficient as it directly targets the affected site. Intranasal solutions can be utilized as a sinus rinse, nose spray, or nebulizer solution depending on the needs of the patient.

Injectable Preparations

Intravenous (IV), intramuscular (IM), and subcutaneous (SQ) compounded medications require additional training and the appropriate facilities to prepare. All of these dosage forms have the potential to be prepared as a solution, and IM and SQ medications can also be prepared as a suspension or emulsion. The only emulsion that is generally given IV in patients is injectable lipid products such as propofol. Outlined previously, solutions are homogenous mixtures– the drug is fully dissolved in the medium – and suspensions are heterogeneous mixtures where the liquid vehicle contains fine amounts of drug distributed throughout. Any injectable medication that is a suspension requires being shaken prior to use in order to ensure even distribution. As discussed in Chapters 1 and 2, 503a compounding facilities preparing sterile compounds that are not for immediate use should meet the minimum requirements set forth by USP 797. Hospital pharmacists have been preparing IV compounded medications for many years now, and the process still has not been perfected. Due to the time needed to prepare this dosage form and the requirements for sterile preparation, the authors recommend either preparing sterile compounds as needed (e.g. for immediate use) or purchasing injectable compounded medications from a reputable compounding pharmacy. IV and IM dosage forms often require the necessary skillset to administer to a patient appropriately, while clients can be easily trained to administer SQ dosage forms.

Ophthalmic Preparations

Ophthalmic compounded medications require additional training and the appropriate facilities to prepare. They are sterile preparations that are instilled into the eye and can be compounded into solutions, suspensions, or ointments. The dosage form utilized is often dependent on the patient's therapeutic needs and which drugs are being utilized. Due to the requirements for sterile preparation, the authors recommend utilizing multiple available manufactured products or prescribing ophthalmic compounded medications from a reputable compounding pharmacy.

Ingredients

Ingredient Selection

The USP established a step-by-step plan for acquiring appropriate ingredients for compounding when commercial products cannot be used. Compounded medications should always be prepared from manufactured FDA-approved medications when they are available and do not negatively impact the formulation. In the case that there is not an FDA-approved medication, the available medication does not incorporate into compounding formulations appropriately, it contains a toxic excipient, or potency and stability are not maintained, then a bulk chemical can be used according to the chemical grade order below in Table 5.1. Monographs from the USP Compounding Compendium that utilize bulk chemicals are prepared using USP and National Formulary (NF) ingredients and have appropriate stability testing completed [10].

For in-house compounding, the authors recommend only preparing products for which the approved product or a USP/NF-grade API is available and appropriate to use as the active ingredient source. While there are cases when other grades are appropriate, these are often limited and special circumstances that are recommended to be prescribed out through a reliable compounding pharmacy. Substances that cannot be used in compounding should be considered. At the time of writing, the FDA has developed lists for 503a and 503b compounding pharmacies that list bulk drug substances that can as well as cannot be used in compounding [12]. The most current regulatory guidance on bulk chemical compounding should be consulted prior to utilizing bulk chemicals to prepare compounded products.

The FDA encourages compounders to be cognizant of where bulk drug substances are purchased from as they can present risks to patients. In general companies that sell bulk drug will obtain vast amounts of bulk powder API that they test for quality and purity while confirming it is the stated drug. They then repackage the powder, as shown in Figure 5.3, into smaller containers for distribution to compounding facilities for formulation preparation. Throughout the supply chain, it is possible that improper repackaging may occur, oversight may be lacking, or APIs may be labeled incorrectly as most bulk substance is a white powder.

Table 5.1 Chemical grades for compounded medications.

Chemical grade	Characterization	Products	Recommendation
USP/NF/FCC [10]	Meets or exceeds the minimum purity standards set by the United States Pharmacopeia/National Formulary/Food Chemicals Codex	Acceptable for food, drug, or medicinal use	Acceptable for use and recommended source of ingredients for compounding for all preparations
British Pharmacopeia (BP)/Japanese Pharmacopeia (JP)/ European Pharmacopeia (EF) Chemicals	Meets or exceeds the minimum specifications and purity standards set by the applicable Pharmacopeia	Acceptable for food, drug, or medicinal use	Acceptable for use and recommended source of ingredients for compounding for all preparations if USP/NF/ FCC grade isn't available
ACS Reagent Chemicals/Analytical Reagent [10, 11]	Meets or exceeds the minimum purity standards set by the American Chemical Society; Require a purity of equal to or greater than 95%	May be acceptable for food, drug, or medicinal use if above options are not available. Materials do not consider whether any impurity present raises human or animal safety concerns [10]	May be used when components of compendium quality are not obtainable; Use cautiously
Chemically Pure (CP)	Laboratory chemicals of suitable purity that are used for general applications; Quality of the product is not known	Acceptable for noncritical tasks in the laboratory setting *Materials do not consider whether any impurity present raises human or animal safety concerns [10]	May be used when components of compendium quality are not obtainable; Use *very* cautiously

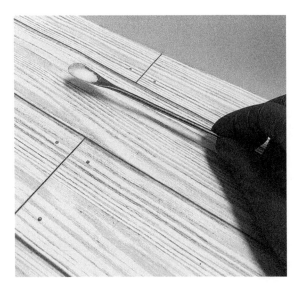

Figure 5.3 Bulk powder on stainless steel spatula.

API repackaging companies may reach out to offer new bulk drug substances they are carrying or lower pricing compared to other repackaging companies. It is the responsibility of the compounder to confirm the quality of the product, if it is legal to compound with, and ensure that it is an appropriate chemical grade. Bulk drug substances are required to be accompanied by a valid certificate of analysis (CoA) and must have been manufactured by an FDA-approved manufacturer in the United States per the Food Drug and Cosmetics Act. For more information, the FDA provides Guidance for Industry: ICHQ7 Good Manufacturing Guidance for APIs as well as a list of warning letters they have issued to API repackaging companies for significant violations of current good manufacturing practice (cGMP) requirements under their "Human Drug Compounding" website link.

A CoA is a piece of documentation that is included with every pharmaceutical ingredient purchased for compounding. The CoA characterizes the ingredients in a product and informs the purchaser what they have paid for. It indicates the allowable range values for that product's assay, which is established by the USP monograph or the manufacturer, and the assay of the specific product that has been purchased. It is the compounder's responsibility to review the CoA and confirm the product is within proper specifications. For any products that fall out of allowable specifications, the compounder must return the product to the manufacturer as this is not considered a "USP-grade" ingredient.

The suppliers of bulk chemical (API) should provide a CoA for each product to the purchaser. If a CoA is not received, then the compounder can contact the manufacturer for it. Sometimes, CoAs will be available to access on the supplier's website in lieu of providing a hard copy. The compounder can also make a blanket request to have the CoA provided with every product if this becomes a nuisance. Upon receiving the CoA, it should be reviewed for the following components:

– Chemical name and Chemical Abstracts Service (CAS) number
– Chemical description
– Chemical assay
– Quantity of water, also known as water of hydration or loss on drying (LOD)

The CAS will always identify the specific chemical formula of the product and is important because it is possible that the chemical name provided may not include the specific salt or ester of the chemical. This can affect a compounded preparation significantly. A comparison should also be made between the CoA chemical description and the characteristics of the product received. Proper comparison can provide a sense of security if the manufacturer's drug source has changed leading to the chemical received having different characteristics than usual, such as color. The chemical assay is discussed above but note that some products have different unit designations and most chemical's activity is provided on a "dry basis." More information regarding assays can be found in Chapter 6. The quantity of water in a chemical is expressed as a percentage and typically coined as LOD. An LOD of 5% informs the compounder that out of 100 mg of product, 5 mg is actually water. If a chemical is stored incorrectly or the container is not closed properly, then the LOD may increase over time and cause a decrease in potency. Incorrect storage also includes leaving powder out in a mortar overnight, as shown in Figure 5.4, as moisture will be absorbed and have a negative effect the compounded preparation.

Solubility

Solubility is the ability of a drug to be dissolved in an aqueous medium. It is measured by the amount of solvent it takes to dissolve 1 g of drug. The solubility of the API that will be incorporated into a compounded preparation will determine the appropriate vehicle and any excipients needed. If a drug

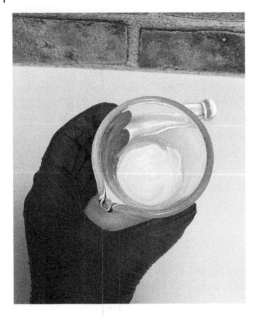

Figure 5.4 Bulk powder in mortar.

has poor aqueous solubility, then the absorption rate will be slower, which may affect bioavailability and the overall effectiveness of the drug. Therefore, improper drug solubility can have one of the biggest impacts on plasma drug concentration achieved and should be accounted for accordingly.

When considering solubility, a solution is formed with a solute(s) and solvent(s). The solute is the substance that is being dissolved, whereas the solvent is the dissolving medium. The definitions of what constitutes being soluble are [13]:

- Very Soluble: Requires **less than 1 part** of solvent for 1 part of solute
- Soluble: Requires **10–30 parts** of solvent for 1 part of solute
- Slightly Soluble: Requires **100–1000 parts** of solvent for 1 part of solute
- Practically Insoluble/Insoluble: Requires **more than 10 000 parts** of solvent for 1 part of solute

Solubility information can often be found in the FDA-approved label of a drug product and provide a general idea of drug solubility. If the package insert contains this information, it will be in the "Description" section of the Drug Label Information. USP has a *Description and Relative Solubility of USP and NF Articles* reference table, but this is usually based on what can be found within the FDA-approved label. The National Library of Medicine has a resource called PubChem (https://pubchem.ncbi.nlm.nih.gov) that allows the user to search any drug and provides a compound summary which includes solubility information under both the "Melting Point" and "Solubility" subheadings.

Partition Coefficient

The partition coefficient is a concept similar to solubility; however, instead of looking at the amount of solute that can be dissolved into a single solvent, partition describes how a solute is distributed between two immiscible solvents [14, 15]. Typically, these solvents are water and octanol, and this process helps predict the hydrophobicity of a drug, which is expressed as the logP.

DrugBank Online (https://go.drugbank.com) is a database that contains a variety of information pertaining to pharmaceutical properties including the logP. This reference and others are summarized in Table 5.11. Each drug has a partition coefficient, or logP, that describes how well it will dissolve in water or an organic solvent which corresponds to the drug's intrinsic properties [16]. A logP value <2, including negative numbers, is indicative of a drug that prefers water or is hydrophilic [17]. A logP value ≥2 is indicative of a drug that prefers octanol or is lipophilic [17].

Hydrophilic drugs are those that dissolve or mix well with water or an aqueous solution. Lipophilic drugs are those that dissolve or mix well with oil. Examples of vehicles that are utilized for aqueous compounds include reverse osmosis (RO) water, suspending agents like Ora-Plus and SUSPENDIT®, and syrups. Examples of oil-based vehicles utilized for nonaqueous medications are olive oil, corn oil, fixed oil, and coconut oil.

A partition coefficient is beneficial for estimating the distribution of a drug within the body. An example of when it would be important is if a client is having trouble giving a cat oral medication. Knowing the partition coefficient of the drug would allow the compounder to determine the feasibility of developing a transdermal product for administration and the expected bioavailability compared to the oral product.

Density

The density of the active ingredient(s) and excipients can affect the uniformity of the mixture. Density relates to how compact a substance is and explains why 1 g of lactose may not visually appear to be the same amount as 1 g of active ingredient (gabapentin, prednisolone, etc.). Powders with a higher density will fall to the bottom of the mixture and those with a lower density rise. This supports the use of geometric dilution when mixing powders as it is very unlikely that you will be mixing ingredients that all have the same density in compounded formulations.

Water Activity

All chemicals have a different degree of hydration or the amount of water molecules they contain. Water activity describes the amount of available water that is present in a nonsterile drug product. Drugs with higher water activity are more likely to support the growth of microorganisms as they provide an appropriate environment for proliferation. High water activity can also increase the rate of chemical degradative reactions. Water activity can range from 0.00 to 1.00, indicating that there is no water activity present or the product is pure water, respectively. The USP differentiates between aqueous and nonaqueous products using a water activity of 0.6. If the product has a water activity of ≥0.6, then it is considered to be aqueous, whereas products with a water activity of <0.6 are termed nonaqueous.

USP <1112> provides a table of water activity information that can be used to develop compounding formulations and determine BUDs and storage requirements.

pH

For liquid formulations, the pH of the drug – and in turn the solubility, stability, and tolerability – is a critical factor [18]. If there is a difference in the pH between the solution of drug and the final compounded preparation, the drug will likely fall out of solution or precipitate. Another important factor to take into consideration is a manufactured solution that is used as part of the compounded product may contain buffers, which can affect the pH of the final product and lead to faster degradation. The best way to prevent a formulation from degrading faster than anticipated is to determine which pH range is most susceptible to degradation for the API.

In the event that the pH of the product is out of range for maintaining stability, buffers can be prepared to maintain the pH of the preparation for its expected BUD. Common buffers that have been used in commercial and compounded products include acetic acid + sodium acetate, ammonia + ammonium chloride, and citric acid + sodium citrate. Limitations with buffers include shifts in pH with temperature change, effects on crystallization, increased pain upon injection, and destabilization with lyophilization. The addition of a base (alkalizing) or an acid (acidifying) can also be utilized and may be preferred over the use of buffers as it minimizes the chance for reduced drug solubility. Alkalinizing agents include sodium hydroxide, sodium bicarbonate, and potassium hydroxide and are used in a formulation to increase the pH. Acidifying agents include acetic acid, citric acid, and tartaric acid and are used in a formulation to decrease the pH.

Mixing a weak acid and its conjugate base, or weak base and its conjugate acid, with water forms a buffer solution. The pH for the entire system that a buffer solution is placed in will be maintained, while an alkalinizing or acidifying agent is added to an acidic or basic solution, which it will modify and maintain. Buffer solutions work by utilizing the formation of an equilibrium between the acid component and conjugate base of the preparation. Through adding the buffer solution, the corresponding conjugate acid or base is provided, stabilizing pH. A buffer solution is an aqueous solution and, therefore, should not be utilized in formulations with nonaqueous vehicles. Buffer solutions only work well for a limited amount of time when added to a strong acid or strong base. The solute will react until it is no longer available, meaning that the solution is no longer a buffer; then, changes in pH can once again occur. The acidifying and alkalinizing agents themselves can be added to any formulation.

Overall, buffer solutions are not ideal for products that have extended BUDs as they can dissipate as well as allow for bacterial growth due to the solution being water based. Acidifying and alkalizing agents neutralize the pH of the system and are preferred for products with longer BUDs as well as nonaqueous preparations.

Chelators

The stability of compounded formulations can be affected by trace metals, such as copper, iron, calcium, and manganese, that are present within formulation components, including the API, excipients, and dispensing container. Chelators are especially problematic when compounding drugs that oxidize easily, a common phenomenon as oxidation is the second most common degradation pathway [19]. Chelating agents are added into a formulation to bind these trace metals and form water-soluble complexes that are inert. Overall, chelating agents minimize the rate of drug degradation and examples of chelators are ascorbic acid, citric acid, glucuronic acid, and saccharic acid. The majority of chelators are soluble in water and alcohol and overlap with antioxidants; therefore, one agent should be used for both functions if possible.

Antioxidants

Antioxidants are utilized in compounding formulations to extend the BUD by delaying or preventing oxidation. The antioxidant effect seen will be dependent on the proclivity of oxidation of the ingredients used in the formula. Oxidation can present itself as a change in color of the preparation, change in taste of the preparation, change in smell of the preparation, or a variety of other changes in appearance. While chelators bind agents that can lead to oxidation forming insoluble complexes, antioxidants provide electrons and hydrogen atoms to reactive species that would otherwise enhance oxidation and in turn drug degradation. These reactive species are free radicals that have partially oxidized intermediates and will trap an electron from any other molecule they can find to compensate for the deficient electron. Examples of antioxidants include acetylcysteine, ascorbic acid, glutathione, and sodium thiosulfate. The compounder should confirm that the antioxidant they select is soluble in the solvent being used for the compounded formulation.

Preservatives

Preservatives are excipients that are added to formulations and have two main benefits for their utilization in compounded formulations. They help protect compounds from chemical change, similar to antioxidants and chelating agents, while also preventing microbial growth. Preservatives are found in most manufactured medications unless they are single-dose or preservative-free injectables. Compounded formulations with aqueous vehicles are more prone to microbial growth than nonaqueous vehicles, which is why it is commonly recommended to refrigerate aqueous preparations if there is not stability data supporting room temperature storage.

Preservatives interfere with various processes within microbial cells, leading to cell damage or death. Formulations may contain more than one preservative as studies have proven that they can act synergistically to enhance their antimicrobial action. Though they are noted as excipients, preservatives are definitely not inactive ingredients, and the concentration included in a formulation cannot be at a toxic level. The ideal concentration for a preservative is high enough to prevent microbial growth without causing toxicity in the patient. The decision of which preservative to add into a formulation can be dependent upon the pH of the drug. Bacterial growth is stunted outside of the pH range of 6–8.4, but the formulation may require a pH within that range in order to prevent drug degradation. For a single preservative, there may be a different pH that inhibits bacterial growth as compared to fungal growth.

The preservative selected for a compounding formulation must also play nice with the active ingredient(s) and other excipients. There is always potential for chemical instability to occur, which is not always represented visually. Preservatives also have the potential to interact with the container system used and can affect product stability. Potential incompatibilities that may occur include the formation of complexes, precipitation of an ingredient, or adsorption. The following interactions/incompatibilities are well documented and should be avoided.

- In the presence of strong oxidizing agents, components can experience incompatibilities.
- Interactions can occur between a strong base and acidic preservatives.
- Cationic preservatives and anionic surfactants are incompatible.
- Nonionic surfactants (polysorbate 80) are incompatible with *some* alcoholic phenolic preservatives.
- Polyvalent cations experience interactions with sorbic acid, butylated hydroxyanisole, and chlorhexidine.

As previously mentioned, preservatives can be toxic not only to microbial cells but to human cells as well. Parenteral products containing benzyl alcohol are contraindicated for neonates due to the association with central nervous system (CNS) effects, cardiovascular failure, and hematological abnormalities. Paraben preservatives are considered irritants and must not be included in ophthalmic medications. Another benzene product, benzalkonium chloride, should not be administered via the ophthalmic route in individuals wearing contacts. Later in this chapter, toxic excipients are noted in Table 5.4, and both benzyl alcohol and benzalkonium chloride are included as potential toxic substances for cats and dogs. Selected preservatives, their appropriate concentration, and their optimal pH are listed in Table 5.2.

Flavors, Coating Agents, and Sweeteners

As most drugs interfere with physiological processes within cells, animals have evolved to sense bitter taste in order to avoid certain compounds. Bitter flavoring is notable with toxic substances and is a deterrent against ingestion. Preparing medications in oral solid dosage forms, such as capsules or coated tablets, can help mask bitter taste. Coating agents are excipients used to coat a dosage carrier (e.g. tablet) to help mask a bitter medication. An additional benefit is coatings work to protect the drug from light and humidity. They may also be utilized to carry the medication to a particular site within the GI tract. Unfortunately, it becomes much harder to mask bitter taste for oral liquid dosage forms. A benefit of compounding is that it allows for the inclusion of flavors and sweeteners to improve compliance for patients. However, flavors have the potential to effect compounded preparations and can lead to drug degradation, therefore the compounder should reference current USP standards to ensure compliance.

Flavors such as maple, marshmallow, mint, coffee, vanilla, and orange have been noted to mask or overcome the unpleasant taste of moderately bitter drugs. Some flavors like coffee complement bitter flavoring and may work well in certain species. More information on species specific flavoring is discussed in Chapter 6. If the addition of flavor does not have a large effect on the bitterness

Table 5.2 Preservatives for compounding.

Preservative	Concentration (%)	Optimal pH	Note(s)
Benzalkonium chloride (liquids, emulsions, intranasals, otics)	0.004–0.1	4–10	Ineffective against resistant pseudomonas strains GI irritant when used orally
Benzoic acid (liquids, emulsions, ointments, creams)	0.1–0.3	<4.5	Moderately active against bacteria, fungus, and mold
Benzyl alcohol (liquids, emulsions, ointments, creams)	1–4	<5	Effective against mold and yeasts Better activity against gram (−) bacteria than gram (+) bacteria Incompatible with methylcellulose
Cresol (liquids, emulsions)	0.3–0.5	<9	Moderately active against bacteria Weak activity against mold and yeasts
Methylparaben (liquids, emulsions, ointments, creams, intranasals, otics)	0.02–0.3	4–8	Most effective against mold and yeasts Broad spectrum of activity against bacteria
Propylparaben (liquids, emulsions, ointments/creams, intranasals, otics)	0.01–0.6	4–8	Activity against molds and yeast is better than activity against bacteria
Phenol (liquids, emulsions)	0.2–0.5	<7	Moderately active against bacteria Weak activity against mold and yeasts
Potassium sorbate (liquids, emulsions, ointments/creams)	0.05–2	<6	Mainly antifungal activity Moderately antibacterial
Sodium benzoate (liquids, emulsions, ointments/creams)	0.1–0.5	2–5	Bacteriostatic and antifungal
Sodium propionate (liquids, emulsions)	<1	<5	Bacteriostatic and antifungal
Sorbic acid (liquids, emulsions, ointments/creams)	0.05–0.2	4.5	Mainly antifungal activity Weak antimicrobial activity Works synergistically with glycol

Source: Adapted from Allen et al. (2019).

of the prepared compound, then a sweeting agent may improve taste. It is important to note that sweeteners do not actually suppress bitterness but instead reduce the perception of bitter flavor. As veterinary patients can have very specific palates, the inclusion of bitterness suppressor may also be warranted.

Instead of reducing the perception of bitter flavor, bitterness suppressor physically modifies the formulation by lowering the bitterness level. Bitter drugs have an amine functional group, which is what leads to the terrible taste. The functional group is blocked by a complex in the bitterness suppressor, and a drastic reduction of bitter taste occurs. Bitter suppressor products are available in powder and liquid forms, and the solvent utilized for the compounded formulation determines which product to use. Liquid forms are water soluble and should be used in aqueous solvents where powder forms can be used in either aqueous or oil-based solvents.

Flavors are also available in both liquid and powder form, Figure 5.5, but typically the liquid products are only compatible with aqueous compounds unless they are a flavored oil (e.g. cod oil).

Powder flavors are compatible with both aqueous and nonaqueous compounds. Emulsifiers are available to utilize for the addition of oil-soluble flavors that you want to add to an aqueous vehicle as well as combining water-soluble flavors in nonaqueous vehicles. Underflavoring the compound will not lead to compliance with veterinary patients, and neither will overflavoring the compound. Anecdotally, compounders determine the amount of flavoring to add by calculating 3% of the total volume of the compound and adding that amount in grams (for powdered flavors) and milliliters (for liquid flavors).

Examples of artificial sweeteners that can be utilized include steviol glycosides, acesulfame potassium, and sucralose. Examples of natural sugars are fructose, honey, agave nectar, and molasses. Drugs that are inherently more bitter will require a larger quantity of sweetener. In general, sweeteners are added to the formulation in a quantity of 0.1–1%.

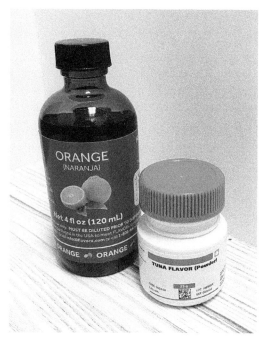

Figure 5.5 Liquid and powdered flavors.

Sodium chloride can also be added to bitter compounds. It is the opposite of bitterness and, therefore, can help reduce bitter flavor and enhance sweetness. Sodium chloride is added in larger amounts (e.g. 0.5–1%) than sweeteners are to formulations.

Coloring Agents

Coloring agents are not necessary for the majority of compounded formulations in veterinary medicine. In human medicine, colored medications have been noted to increase compliance in children, but this is not applicable for animal patients with the potential exception of birds. Coloring agents are most beneficial when used as tracers to ensure the homogeneity of powders combined for compounding capsules or powders. They should be purchased in powder form for this use and be specifically approved for the use in food, drugs, and cosmetics. These products will be indicated by the notation FD&C (Federal Food, Drug and Cosmetic Act) in front of the colorant name and number [20]. Some vitamin powders such as cyanocobalamin and riboflavin are brightly colored and can be used as tracers without using synthetic coloring. The use of tracers will be discussed further in Chapter 6 with geometric dilution.

Salt Forms

The form and purity of each ingredient has to be taken into account when developing a compounding formulation. The form of a drug is present on the manufacturer's package insert, if utilizing an FDA-approved product, or on the USP monograph, if utilizing a bulk drug. The CoA provides additional information about the drug. Drugs that are in salt form do not contain 100% active drug, and the compounder must be aware of this when completing compounding calculations. An example of this is dexamethasone sodium phosphate injection labeled as 4 mg/ml but that includes the weight of the sodium phosphate, so this product actually only contains 3 mg/ml of dexamethasone. Salt form holds a high importance in compounding as around 50%

of FDA approvals of APIs are in the salt form [21]. If the salt form can have a detrimental effect on compounding calculations, why would we use it?

– Salt forms can augment the state of a drug.
– Salt forms can increase aqueous solubility of a drug.
– Salt forms can stabilize the polymorph, or crystalline structure, of a drug.
– Salt forms can increase the dissolution rate of a drug.

Often if a drug is a weak acid or weak base, its salt form will be used to increase the drug's limited water solubility. However, as increased solubility leads to faster dissolution, the drug would begin dissolving in the mouth and lead to a bitter taste. One salt form in particular, stearic acid, has reduced solubility and is utilized in suspensions to help suppress bitter taste [21]. Drugs in salt form are not nearly as stable either. Some salt forms have been shown to interact with excipients, which can affect the integrity of the compounded formulation. If there is not a USP monograph available or stability study, appropriate research needs to be completed to confirm that no interactions will occur.

Salts placed in an aqueous environment may not completely dissolve. The dissolution is dependent upon the pH of the environment they are placed in as well as the aqueous solubility of the salt form. The part that dissolves will contain both ionized and unionized components. Recall from pharmacology that only unionized drug is able to be systemically absorbed and ultimately have an effect on the body. This reaction is described by the drug's pKa and the pH of the environment.

USP does not outline whether the compounder must complete their calculations using the base form of the drug or the salt form. It is up to the compounder to utilize their clinical knowledge and the information provided in the package insert from the manufacturer, the USP monograph, and/or the CoA to determine their routine procedure. A standard operating procedure (SOP) should be developed with regard to this process and notate if there are any drugs that deviate from the standard protocol. An example of making this distinction is with metronidazole. Metronidazole base naturally has an extremely bitter taste, but its salt form, metronidazole benzoate, is far more palatable. Metronidazole base is more potent than metronidazole benzoate with 1 mg of metronidazole base being equivalent to 1.6 mg of metronidazole benzoate. The compounder must be clear on which form of metronidazole they are using for the compounding formula, or the patient may be over- or underdosed.

Organic Salts

Organic salt forms are often used to enhance the solubility of drugs that are insoluble, but they can also be incorporated into drugs to allow for the development of other dosage forms. Organic salts contain covalent carbon–hydrogen bonds, which require less energy to break and, therefore, are generally weaker. Medications that have been combined with a salt to produce an organic salt form include atropine sulfate, butorphanol tartrate, ephedrine sulfate, and phenylephrine hydrochloride.

Inorganic Salts

Inorganic salt forms are more challenging as they can undergo physical and chemical changes during the compounding process. Factors that can affect the properties of inorganic salts include particle size, pH, and water content [21]. Regarding water content, the powder can absorb moisture from the air or water can evaporate from the powder. This may cause inconsistencies when weighing out powders that can lead to the compounded formulation not being within the expected ±10% range. Inorganic salts contain ionic bonds and do not contain both carbon and hydrogen like their organic salt counterparts. Ionic bonds require more energy to break and, therefore, are more stable. Examples of inorganic salts include sodium chloride, calcium chloride, sodium bicarbonate, and calcium carbonate.

Common Excipients by Dosage Form
Compounding formulations often require the incorporation of suitable inactive ingredients, or excipients, to work appropriately. Excipients do not directly provide therapeutic activity for the compound. They can however:

– Promote proper incorporation of the API
– Maintain pH of the compound
– Prevent the API from settling into a solid mass or cake
– Protect the API from degradation
– Preserve stability of the compound over an extended period of time
– Increase patient palatability or aid in medication administration
– Promote enhanced drug delivery

Determining the solvent to utilize for a compounded medication requires an understanding of the API. Table 5.3 summarizes the most common excipients used in compounding nonsterile products, their purpose for being used in a compounding formulation, and selected examples of products classified under each excipient type. Acquiring a foundational knowledge regarding excipients is important as they may be your formulation's saving grace, or they may adversely alter the bioavailability or absorption of your compound.

Compounding formulations may utilize premade bases to ease the compounding process and create more consistent products. Premade bases contain a variety of excipients that prevent bacterial growth, increase palatability, and prevent phase one reactions (hydrolysis, oxidation, etc.). Upon inspection of any premade base that is ordered and received, it can be noted that the expiration dates are in line with manufactured drugs. This is because they are FDA-approved products that have undergone the appropriate testing and approval process. Prior to substituting or including any premade base in a compounding formulation, the ingredient list must be reviewed to confirm that there will not be any interactions with the active ingredient(s) or other excipients. All premade bases will include a preservative, at the least, requiring the compounder to confirm that there will not be any product or container incompatibilities.

Oral Liquid Medications

Excipients utilized for oral liquid medications include solvent(s) that are used to dissolve the API, flavoring, and sweeteners to enhance the palatability, preservatives to assist in preventing microbial growth, suspending agents, and antioxidants and chelators, which are grouped together as stabilizers, to assist in preventing drug degradation.

Oral Solid Medications

Excipients utilized for oral solid medications differ between capsules and tablets. Capsules typically require a diluent or filler to alter the strength of the medication while providing additional bulk that makes it easier to work with. Tablets may use an assortment of excipients, such as

Table 5.3 Excipients for nonsterile compounding.

Excipient	Functionality	Example(s)
Antioxidant	Minimize oxidation	Ascorbic acid, vitamin E, BHA
Base	Holds API; increases delivery for topical preparations	VersaPro™, Lipoderm, Mucolox™, Pluronic Lecithin Organogel (PLO)
Binder	Hold ingredients together	Lactose monohydrate, microcrystalline cellulose, sucrose powder
Capsule	Enclose ingredient(s)	Hard shell (gel), soft shell
Chelating agent	Stabilize dosage form	EDTA, Citric acid
Coating agent	Mask unpleasant taste	Wax, lipid, microcrystalline cellulose, latex, stearic acid
Coloring agent	Improve compliance; Ensure properly mixed	Powder, liquid
Diluent (filler)	Increase dosage size or bulk	Lactose monohydrate, microcrystalline cellulose, calcium carbonate
Disintegrant	Promote release of API	Cellulose, starch
Emollient	Increase absorption (topical)	Lanolin, paraffin, silicone, petrolatum
Flavor	Enhance palatability	Powder, liquid (usually limited to aqueous products)
Glidant/ Anticaking	Reduce clumping	Magnesium stearate, talc, starch
Humectant	Prevent drying	Propylene glycol, glycerin, polyethylene glycol (300)
Levigating agent	Enhance powder incorporation	Propylene glycol, glycerin, ethoxy diglycol
Lubricant	Reduce friction	Stearic acid, hydrogenated vegetable oil, magnesium stearate
pH modifier	Maintain physiologic pH	Citric acid, sodium hydroxide
Plasticizer	Increase flexibility	Propylene glycol, glycerin, polyethylene glycol (200–6000)
Preservative	Prevent/minimize microbial growth	Benzyl alcohol, benzalkonium chloride, sodium benzoate, methylparaben, propylparaben
Solvent/Vehicle	Dissolve/suspend API	RO water, corn oil, simple syrup
Stiffening agent	Increase viscosity/thickness	Hydrogenated castor oil, stearyl alcohol, glyceryl distearate
Surfactant	Reduce surface tension	Stearyl alcohol, lanolin, petrolatum, oleic acid, paraffin wax, beeswax
Suspending agent	Increase dispersion	Acacia, gelatin, agar, hydroxyethyl cellulose, sodium alginate, alginic acid, starch, xanthan gum
Sweetener	Enhance palatability	Sucrose, sorbitol, aspartame, glycerol

diluents or fillers, to increase the amount of powder to work with, binders to adhere the API and other powders together, lubricants to allow for a pharmaceutically elegant product, disintegrating agents that promote the disintegration and therefore dissolution of the compound following administration, and coatings that may control disintegration, improve palatability, or enhance stability.

Emulsions

Excipients utilized for emulsions include surfactants to reduce the surface tension between the oil and water phases allowing for a well-blended product and flavoring to enhance the palatability.

Transdermal Medications

Excipients utilized for transdermal medications include the premade base (e.g. Lipoderm®) or vehicle, which gives the formulation its properties and antioxidants to extend the BUD. When a premade base is not used, additional excipients may be added to the formulation, which include penetration enhancers and preservatives.

Cream, Gel, and Ointment Medications

Excipients utilized for cream, gel, and ointment medications are the base or vehicle that gives the formulation its properties, antioxidants, and chelating agents to extend BUD, stiffening agents to adjust the feel or application of the medication, and buffering agents or acidifying/alkalinizing agents to adjust the pH.

In an ideal world, excipients would be completely inert and nontoxic, but, in practice, this almost never happens. An excipient can be toxic on its own in compounded preparations, especially in high quantities can lead to toxicity after interacting with other excipients or active ingredients, or degradation of the excipient may generate toxic metabolites. Examples of excipients and adverse reactions they have caused are listed in Table 5.4. The addition of excipients to any compounding formulation requires a full understanding of how the excipient may interact with all the other formulation ingredients to guarantee the safety of the patient.

Table 5.4 Examples of excipients and their adverse reactions.

Excipient	Function	Adverse reaction	Species
Benzene ring preservatives (Benzalkonium chloride, Benzyl alcohol)	Preservative	Bronchoconstriction, CNS toxicity, ocular toxicity	Cats[a], dogs[a]
Cremophor EL (polyoxyl 35 castor oil)	Emulsifier, Solubilizing agent, Surfactant	Hypersensitivity (anaphylaxis)	Cats, dogs
Lactose	Filler	Caution in patients with lactase deficiency or galactosaemia	Cats[b], dogs
Lanolin	Emulsifier	Skin hypersensitivity reactions, tremors/seizures (*dogs*)	Cats, dogs[c]
Propylene glycol	Wetting agent	Heinz body anemia	Cats[d]
Sodium metabisulphite	Antioxidant	Hypersensitivity (bronchospasm, anaphylaxis)	Cats, dogs

[a] When ingested in large quantities (e.g. grooming after application of topical products) or injected intravenously.
[b] The use of lactose, clinically, in capsules has been proven safe for cats even with the general assumption that they are lactose intolerant.
[c] When ingested in large quantities (e.g. grooming after application of topical products).
[d] Requires large quantity; Propylene glycol should never be used as a vehicle in compounded preparations for cats.

Hazardous Drugs

As discussed in Chapter 1, the National Institute for Occupational Safety and Health (NIOSH) publishes a list of hazardous drugs that are used in the healthcare setting. Classifications for hazardous drugs can be found in the most recent version of the *NIOSH List of Antineoplastic and Other Hazardous Drugs in Healthcare Settings* publication.

NIOSH criteria define a drug as being hazardous if they exhibit one or more of the following six characteristics in humans or animals: carcinogenicity, teratogenicity or other developmental toxicity, reproductive toxicity, organ toxicity at low doses, genotoxicity, and structure and toxicity profiles of new drugs that mimic existing drugs determined hazardous by the above criteria [22]. USP 800 provides specifications for compounding hazardous drugs and stipulates when nonsterile and sterile compounds must be prepared in a containment primary engineering control in order to reduce hazardous drug exposure. Hazardous drugs that may require compounding include, but are not limited to, apomorphine, methimazole, mycophenolate, phenoxybenzamine, spironolactone, and zonisamide [22]. Therefore, it is important to review USP 800 prior to compounding any medication classified as hazardous by the NIOSH.

The NIOSH list will change with each new publication and, therefore, should be reviewed at least annually and each time a new drug is approved. The site should have a prepared list of any medications that are on the NIOSH list or meet the specifications above. Veterinary only drugs may not be included on the list as it is focused on human healthcare; therefore, the site should confirm that none of their medications mimic the toxicity profiles of an existing hazardous drug. Following a review of USP 800, if the facilities do not meet the requirements, hazardous drugs should not be compounded as this can lead to exposure to all personnel handling them.

Beyond-Use Dates

As discussed in Chapter 3, BUDs indicate for how long a compounded product will maintain appropriate stability without bacterial growth. Aqueous compounds support the growth of bacteria and fungus when they have a water activity ≥0.6 and are more susceptible to degradation via hydrolysis. Water activity is discussed further in USP Chapter <1112>. Preservatives, which help prevent the growth of microbes, should be added to aqueous compounds that are prepared in a nonsterile environment due to the potential for inadvertent contamination. For nonsterile aqueous compounds that cannot contain preservatives, the preparation must be stored under refrigerated temperatures as long as the temperature will not affect the properties of the preparation.

Nonaqueous compounds are those that have a water activity of <0.6 as this does not support the growth of bacteria and fungus. A lower water activity may also limit drug degradation due to decrease hydrolysis. Liquids are more apt to degrade under storage conditions than powders and, therefore, tend to have shorter BUDs. USP has established default dating for nonsterile and sterile compounded products that can be found in <795> and <797>, respectively. If there is not an existing formula available for a compounded product, the compounder can develop their own. After confirming the ingredients to be included in the formula, the BUD should be considered. The reader should refer to the most recently published version of <795> for default dating standards.

If the compounder would like to extend the BUD of the product, they must first complete a stability-indicating assay to prove that the compound will maintain its stability for the intended duration and prevent microbial growth for that time period. In the case that both of these criteria are met, the stability-indicating assay should be kept on file for reference, and the BUD of the product can be extended. If one or both of these criteria are not met, default dating must be used. The exception to this would be if the drug concentration fell out of range or microbial growth occurred prior to the default dating expiration. In this case, the BUD should be adjusted. BUD recommendations are a guideline, and if a problem is noted with a formulation, expected therapeutic concentrations, or expected symptomatic improvement is not observed, the formulation should be reviewed, and the duration of use shortened appropriately.

When developing formulations for in-house compounding, the authors recommend preparing compounds in line with USP monographs if possible as these formulations are clearly defined with BUDs that meet the requirements for stability and microbial growth prevention. If a USP monograph is not available, published stability studies can be referenced. If using published studies, refer to the discussion in Chapter 3 to verify that the referenced study is stability indicating and ensure that microbial growth prevention is sufficient. In these cases, when in doubt if the published study meets the requirements for an extended BUD, use the formulation in the study but utilize the USP default dating instead.

Formulation Resources

The USP Compounding Compendium was created to help ensure the standard and quality of formulations used in both human and animal patients. The Compounding Compendium contains monographs to assist practitioners with nonsterile and sterile compounding when a manufactured product cannot reasonably be used in their patient. The compounded preparation monographs should be the first formulation resource that is utilized by practitioners trying to find an appropriate formula. All the monographs that are available in the USP Compounding Compendium have the appropriate formulas including ingredients and quantities, directions for compounding, BUD based upon stability studies, packaging and storage information, acceptable pH ranges for the ingredient(s), and stability-indicating assays [23]. The USP works to identify formulas that need to be prioritized for development by requesting feedback from clinicians and pharmacists that compound.

In the event that the Compounding Compendium does not have the formulation needed, another option is utilizing the USP BUD default guidelines. When the compounder does not feel comfortable developing their own formulation or requires a longer BUD than the default guidelines provide for the formulation, there are other resources that can be utilized. Books, journals, and websites can provide formulations and formulation development tools. Examples of these are NCBI PubMed, the *International Journal of Pharmaceutical Compounding* (IJPC), Trissel's Stability of Compounding Formulations, and Compounding Today. It is vital to review the formulations found in these resources and their citations thoroughly to determine if they have completed the necessary stability testing to support their stated BUD. The pharmaceutical compounding company that bulk chemicals are purchased through may also provide formulation support, though some require a membership.

Calculations

All the processes in compounding – formulation development, preparation, packaging, dispensation – involve calculations. The calculations must be completed correctly during the development of the formulation as they will be utilized each subsequent time the medication is prepared. It should be guaranteed that the master formula is correct and easily repeatable for future prescriptions. If making multiple strengths of the same compound, a new master formulation should be created for each strength to decrease the risk of calculation errors occurring. Calculations are a significant source of error in both creating and preparing compounded medications but ensuring accurate dosing leaves zero room for error. Familiarity with converting between measurements, such as percentages and grams/milligrams, is advantageous as any error that is made can have severe consequences for your patient(s). It is also advisable to setup formulation documentation to walk someone step by step through the math for the compound. See Figures 5.6 and 5.7 for examples of this.

Product: ABC Drug Suspension 20 mg/ml BUD: 90 days Qty: [ ] ml

100 ml Minimum
50 ml Increments

Date __/__/__ Lot: ________ Exp: __/__/__

Product/Ingredients	Quantity
ABC drug powder NDC: ______ Lot: Exp: Mfr:	
RO water	Small amount
Simple syrup NDC: ______ Lot: Exp: Mfr:	QS to [ ] ml

[ ] = Total ml

ABC drug powder	(Total) ml × 2 g / 100 ml = ABC drug powder g	([ ]) ml × 2 g / 100 ml = _____ g
RO water	Just enough to make a paste	Small amount
Simple syrup	QS to (Total) ml	QS to [ ] ml

Figure 5.6 Example formulation record sheet ingredient calculations for an oral suspension. The quantity to be made is placed into each gray box and then the calculations are completed as written.

Product: ABC Drug/XYZ Drug Otic (2:1) BUD: 30 days Qty [ ] ml

5 ml Minimum
5 ml Increments

Date __/__/__ Lot: ________ Exp: __/__/__

Product/Ingredients	Quantity
ABC drug NDC: ______ Lot: Exp: Mfr:	
XYZ drug NDC: ______ Lot: Exp: Mfr:	

[ ] = Total ml

ABC drug	(Total) ml / 5 × 3.3 = ABC drug ml	[ ] ml / 5 × 3.3 = _____ ml
XYZ drug	(Total) ml / 5 × 1.7 = XYZ drug ml	[ ] ml / 5 × 1.7 = _____ ml

Figure 5.7 Example formulation record sheet ingredient calculations for an otic solution prepared from two injectable solutions. The quantity to be made is placed into each gray box and then the calculations are completed as written.

Errors have the potential to occur when selecting the appropriate products and weighing out or drawing up the ingredients for a compound. They can also occur when diluting medications or converting the volume of liquid to a weight (w/v ➜ w/w) or the inverse. Confirm that the scale being utilized is appropriately calibrated and those who may prepare compounded medications know how to use it. A torsion balance can be used as long as the least weighable quantity (LWQ) is determined to confirm the sensitivity of the balance. The LWQ can only be determined if the compounder knows the sensitivity requirement and acceptable error for the torsion balance. Sensitivity requirement is the weight (in milligrams) that can be added or removed before the dial moves one division. In general, torsion balances have a sensitivity requirement of 6 mg. The percentage of acceptable error is the allowable error that you have noted in your SOP for compounded preparations, which is generally 5%. When weighing a capsule that should weigh 100 mg, a 5% acceptable error allows the capsule to range from 95 to 105 mg. Torsion balances and other equipment are more thoroughly discussed in Chapter 6.

Refer to Table 5.5 for equations for LWQ, dilution, ratio, w/v, and v/v as well as examples for each and to Table 5.6 for drug concentration conversions.

Table 5.5 Compounding equations and examples.

Equation	Use example
$LWQ = 100\% * \dfrac{\left(Sensivity\ \mathrm{Re}quirement\ in\,mg\right)}{Acceptable\ Error\ in\%}$	If you have a scale with a sensitivity requirement of 6 mg and your acceptable error is 5%, then the LWQ is 120 mg. You can see in the below equation, that the percentage units cancel out leaving your final answer in mg. $LWQ = 100\% * \dfrac{6mg}{5\%}$
Dilution = Part (solvent): Whole (*solution*)	You want to prepare a 1:10 ketamine dilution for a CRI, and you have 1 ml of ketamine to dilute. This means you have **1 ml of ketamine** and **9 ml of diluent** which makes a **total of 10 ml** when combined. 1:10 solution = 1 part drug: 10 parts total solution = 9 parts diluent
Ratio = Part (solute): Part (*solvent*)	You want to prepare a 1:10 ketamine to diluent ratio for a CRI, and you have 1 ml of ketamine to dilute. This means you have **1 ml of ketamine** and **10 ml of diluent** which makes a **total of 11 ml** when combined. 1:10 = 1 part drug to 10 parts diluent = 11 parts total solution OR 1:11 dilution
w/v = mg/ml; g/ml; g/l	Liquid medications are expressed in w/v such as mg/ml. Your ketamine in the above example is an example since the concentration is 100 mg/ml.
w/w = mg/mg; mg/g; gm/g; mcg/mg	Nonliquid medications such as creams and some pastes are expressed as w/w because the total volume is expressed as weight instead of volume. A cream that is 30 mg/g would be 30 mg of drug in every 1 g of cream.

Table 5.6 Drug concentration conversions.

(x)%	g/ml	mg/ml	(x) : (y)
10% solution	10 g/100 ml solution	100 mg/ml	1 : 10
1% solution	1 g/100 ml solution	10 mg/ml	1 : 100
0.1% solution	0.1 g/100 ml	1 mg/ml	1 : 1000
0.01% solution	0.01 g/100 ml	0.1 mg/ml	1 : 10 000

Measurements Used in Compounding

The process of compounding employs measurements from several different systems including the metric system, the apothecary system, the avoirdupois system, and the common household system (e.g. cooking). The conversions between these systems and primary nomenclature are shown in Tables 5.7 and 5.8. A general understanding of nomenclature and equivalents between the measurement systems will increase comfort with compounding, prevent errors, and save the compounder time. When transitioning between units, there are also common pharmacy equivalents that are used and can be found in Table 5.9. Rounding should not be completed until the final answer for the calculation.

Displacement Factor

Not taking the displacement factor into account can significantly change the strength of a compounded formulation. When adding 20 ml of water to 80 ml of water, we know that the volume that results will be 100 ml. However, if we add 5 g of lactose to 95 ml of water, the total volume will end up being greater than 100 ml. This is because 5 g of lactose occupies more space than 5 ml of water does. Powders have their own displacement volumes, and they have to be taken into account. Displacement will occur for solutions in addition to dosage forms where visible powder remains.

Due to displacement factors, many compounded drugs are "Quantum satis" (QS), which means adding as much of the ingredient as needed to achieve the desired result. Often the last ingredient will have a notation that says "QS the solution" indicating that after you have completed the mixing of the other ingredients, you will only measure out enough of the final ingredient to obtain the final expected volume.

In Figure 5.8, the formula will have a total of four other ingredients that can displace the quantity of Solvent X. It is known that 3 ml of flavor will displace 3 ml of the solvent, but we do not know

Table 5.7 Metric equivalents.

Symbol	Prefix	Meaning	Conversion
K	Kilo	One thousand times	Base unit $\times 10^3$
H	Hecto	One hundred times	Base unit $\times 10^2$
D	Deci	One tenth	Base unit $\times 10^{-1}$
C	Centi	One hundredth	Base unit $\times 10^{-2}$
M	Milli	One thousandth	Base unit $\times 10^{-3}$
mcg/μg	Micro	One millionth	Base unit $\times 10^{-6}$

Table 5.8   Other measurement system equivalents.

	System	Unit (Symbol)	Equivalent
Volume	*Apothecary*	Fluidounce (℥)	30 ml
		Pint (pt)	16 ℥ = 480 ml
		Quart (qt)	2 pt = 32 ℥ = 960 ml
		Gallon (gal)	4 qt = 8 pt. = 3840 ml
	Household	Teaspoon (tsp/t)	5 ml
		Tablespoon (tbsp/T)	3 tsp = 15 ml
		Fluid ounce (fl oz)	2 tbsp = 30 ml
		Cup (c)	8 fl oz
		Pint (pt)	2 c = 480 ml
		Quart (qt)	2 pt = 4 c = 960 ml
		Gallon (gal)	4 qt = 16 c = 3840 ml
Weight	*Avoirdupois*	Grain (gr)	65 mg
		Ounce (oz)	473.5 gr = 30 g
		Pound (lb)	16 oz = 7000 gr = 454 g
	Apothecary	Grain (gr)	65 mg
		Scruple (℈)	20 gr = 1.3 g
		Dram (ℨ)	3 ℈ = 60 gr = 3.9 g
		Ounce (℥)	8 ℨ = 480 gr = 30 g
		Pound (#)	12 ℥ = 5760 gr = 373.2 g
	Household	Ounce (oz)	30 g
		Pound (lb)	16 oz = 454 g

Table 5.9   Common pharmacy equivalents.

1 pt = 473 ml	1 mg = 1000 mcg
1 g = 15.432 gr	1 g = 1000 mg
1 gr = 64.8 mg	1 kg = 1000 g
1 oz = 28.35 g	1 in = 2.54 cm
1 kg = 2.2 lb	1 cm = 0.394 in

Figure 5.8   Example QS compounding formula.

Drug X 5% Formula

Drug X = 5 grams

Excipient A = 0.05 mg

Excipient B = 1 mg

Flavor A = 3 ml

Solvent X = QS 100 ml

how much volume Drug X, Excipient A, and Excipient B will displace. That is why we would QS a formulation, ensuring that the strength desired is prepared. Chapter 6 will cover appropriate techniques for accurately QS-ing a compound.

Capsules: Packing Statistics

For the preparation of capsules, it is necessary to complete packing statistics to determine the volume of the capsule that will be filled by each ingredient. Regardless of whether capsules are prepared by hand-packing or with a capsule machine, the assumption that all capsules will be filled completely allows for the assumption that the correct amount of active drug will be in each capsule. Packing statistics are essential for these assumptions to be true.

The API and filler that are being utilized will be needed to complete this step. Lactose is a common filler used in compounding. It is important to understand that any time the supplier of any ingredient changes or a new lot number is used, packing statistics will need redone. Each ingredient being incorporated into the capsule will need to have its packing statistics determined. Follow the process below to complete packing statistics for capsules that are hand-packed or made utilizing a capsule machine. Figures 5.9 and 5.10 provide example capsule formula worksheets.

Packing Statistic of Drug

Average Weight of Ingredients

1) Weigh out 10 empty capsules (including both the top and bottom) and then divide the total weight by 10 in order to determine the average capsule weight.
2) Utilize bulk chemical, crushed tablets, or capsule contents and fill an appropriately sized weigh boat.
3) Firmly press the bottom of the capsule into the powder while using a twisting motion to fill it completely. This may require picking up the capsule and moving repeatedly to ensure that it is completely filled.
4) Place the top of the capsule onto the bottom of the capsule that is full of powder and then repeat this process for four additional capsules (for a total of five filled capsules).
5) Weigh each individual capsule and record the weight.
6) Subtract the average weight of the empty capsule (determined in step 1) from each recorded weight of the filled capsules (determined in step 5).
7) Calculate your average weight of a capsule by adding the five weights (determined in step 6) and divide by 5.

Percentage of Drug per Capsule Using Bulk Powder

1) Subtract the weight of an empty capsule from the average weight when filled with drug to determine the packing statistic of the drug.
2) To determine the amount of API per capsule, divide the desired strength of the product by the packing statistic of drug and multiply it by 100.
   a) This is the percent of drug per capsule.

Capsule Formula worksheet

Product _____ Date _____/_____/_____

QTY Calculated _____   Strength [＿＿＿＿＿＿]

Gather drug powder, lactose and appropriately sized empty gel caps
Count 50 empty gel caps and weigh, enter in the table below.
Tape off half of the holes in the 100ct capsule machine. Place 50 capsules in the machine and remove tops as usual. Fill cap bottoms with drug powder and tamp until full. Replace tops and remove capsules. Weigh all 50 and record in the table below then convert from grams to milligrams. Repeat for Lactose, then convert from grams to milligrams.

Product/Ingredients	Average weights	
$\dfrac{50 \text{ empty caps total wt}}{50}$ = Average empty capsule weight gm × 1000 = mg	[＿＿＿] / 50 = _____ gm × 1000 = [＿＿＿]	Average empty capsule weight in mg
$\dfrac{50 \text{ Drug caps total wt}}{50}$ = Average drug capsule weight gm × 1000 = mg	[＿＿＿] / 50 = _____ gm × 1000 = [＿＿＿]	Average drug filled capsule weight in mg.
$\dfrac{50 \text{ Lactose caps total wt}}{50}$ = Average lactose capsule weight gm × 1000 = mg	[＿＿＿] / 50 = _____ gm × 1000 = [＿＿＿]	Average Lactose Filled capsule weight in mg.

Determine Packing stat of drug
[＿＿＿] − [＿＿＿] = [＿＿＿] mg Packing Stat of drug   Drug Average full capsule weight mg   Average empty capsule weight gm

Determine percent of drug per capsule:
$\dfrac{\text{Desired Strength of capsule}}{\text{Packing stat of drug}}$ × 100 = % of drug per capsule $\dfrac{[\quad]}{[\quad]}$ × 100 = [＿＿＿] % of drug per capsule

Determine Packing stat of Lactose
[＿＿＿] − [＿＿＿] = [＿＿＿] mg Packing Stat of Lactose   **Average Lactose filled capsule weight**   Average empty capsule weight

Determine Lactose Weight		
100% - % drug per capsule = % of Lactose needed	100% - [＿＿＿] = [＿＿＿]	% of Lactose
$\dfrac{\% \text{ Lactose needed × Lactose Packing Stat}}{100}$ = mg of Lactose	$\dfrac{[\quad] \times [\quad]}{100}$ = [＿＿＿] mg of Lactose	
Convert mg to gm		
$\dfrac{\text{Strength × 100 Capsules}}{1000}$ = **Drug** gm	$\dfrac{[\quad] \times 100 \text{ Capsules}}{1000}$ = _____ gm	
$\dfrac{\text{Lactose mg × 100 Capsules}}{1000}$ = **Lactose** gm	$\dfrac{[\quad] \times 100 \text{ Capsules}}{1000}$ = _____ gm	

Figure 5.9   Capsule formula worksheet for using bulk powder as the drug source.

Percentage of Drug per Capsule Using Manufactured Tablet

1) Subtract the weight of an empty capsule from the average weight when filled with drug to determine the packing statistic of the drug.
2) To determine the weight of manufactured drug per capsule/tablet, divide the total mg in the commercial dosage unit by the total weight of the commercial unit.
3) Then, divide the desired strength of the capsule by the answer from Step 2.
   a) This is the weight of the manufactured drug per capsule.

Capsule Formula worksheet

Product _____   Date _____/_____/_____

QTY Calculated _____   Strength [   ]

Gather drug powder, lactose and appropriately sized empty gel caps
Count 50 empty gel caps and weigh, enter in the table below.
Tape off half of the holes in the 100ct capsule machine. Place 50 capsules in the machine and remove tops as usual. Fill cap bottoms with drug powder and tamp until full. Replace tops and remove capsules. Weigh all 50 and record in the table below then convert from grams to milligrams. Repeat for Lactose, then convert from grams to milligrams.

Product/Ingredients	Average weights		
$\dfrac{50 \text{ empty caps wt}}{50} = \dfrac{\text{Average cap}}{\text{weight gm}}$ × 1000 = mg	$\dfrac{[\quad]}{50}$ = _____ gm × 1000 = [ ]		Average cap weight in mg.
$\dfrac{50 \text{ Drug caps total wt}}{50} = \dfrac{\text{Average drug}}{\text{capsule weight gm}}$ × 1000 = mg	$\dfrac{[\quad]}{50}$ = _____ gm × 1000 = [ ]		Average drug filled capsule weight in mg.
$\dfrac{50 \text{ Lactose caps total wt}}{50} = \dfrac{\text{Average lactose}}{\text{capsule weight gm}}$ × 1000 = mg	$\dfrac{[\quad]}{50}$ = _____ gm × 1000 = [ ]		Average Lactose Filled capsule weight in mg.

Determine Packing stat of drug

[   ] − [   ] = [   ] mg Packing Stat of drug

Drug Average full   Average cap
capsule weight mg   weight mg*

Determine weight of manufactured drug **per capsule:**

$\dfrac{\text{Desired Strength of capsule}}{X} = \dfrac{\text{Total mg in commercial dosage unit}}{\text{Total weight of commercial dosage unit}}$ $\dfrac{[\quad]}{[\quad]} = [\quad]$

Determine percent of drug **per capsule:**

$\dfrac{\text{Weight of Manufactured drug per cap}}{\text{Packing stat of drug}}$ × 100 = % of drug per capsule $\dfrac{[\quad]}{[\quad]}$ × 100 = [   ] % of drug per capsule

Determine Packing stat of Lactose

[   ] − [   ] = [   ] mg Packing Stat of Lactose

Average Lactose   Average empty
filled capsule weight   capsule weight

Determine Lactose Weight

100% - % drug per capsule = % of Lactose needed	100% - [ ] = [ ] % of Lactose
$\dfrac{\% \text{ Lactose needed} \times \text{Lactose Packing Stat}}{100}$ = mg of Lactose	$\dfrac{[\quad] \times [\quad]}{100} = [\quad]$ mg of Lactose
Convert mg to gm	
$\dfrac{\text{Manufactured Drug Strength} \times 100 \text{ Capsules}}{1000}$ = **Drug** gm	$\dfrac{[\quad] \times 100 \text{ Capsules}}{1000}$ = _____ gm
$\dfrac{\text{Lactose mg} \times 100 \text{ Capsules}}{1000}$ = **Lactose** gm	$\dfrac{[\quad] \times 100 \text{ Capsules}}{1000}$ = _____ gm

*Alternatively can do $\dfrac{\text{Strength} \times 100 \text{ Capsules}}{\text{Manufactured Drug Strength}}$ = # tablets / capsules

Figure 5.10   Capsule formula worksheet for using manufactured tablet as the drug source.

4) To determine the percent of drug per capsule, divide the weight of manufactured drug per capsule by the packing statistics of the drug and multiple it by 100.
   a) This is the percent of drug per capsule.

Percentage/Amount of Filler per Capsule

1) Follow the same process as above for the average weight of ingredients for your filler.
2) Subtract the weight of an empty capsule from the average weight when filled with filler to determine the packing statistic of the filler.
3) To determine the percent of filler per capsule, subtract the percent of drug per capsule that was calculated above from 100%.
   a) This is the percent of filler per capsule.
4) To determine the weight that the filler will take up, multiply the percent of filler by the filler packing statistic and divide by 100.
   a) This is the milligrams of filler that will be needed per capsule.

Conversion to Grams

1) Multiply the strength of the drug you are intending to compound by the number of capsules you want to compound (100 or 300 are typical when using a capsule machine) and divide by 1000.
   a) This is the amount of drug in grams that you will weigh out.
2) Multiply the milligrams of filler needed per capsule by the number of capsules you want to compound (100 or 300 are typical when using a capsule machine) and divide by 1000.
   a) This is the amount of filler in grams that you will weigh out.

The weighed-out drug and filler will need to be triturated together using geometric dilution. This process involves taking the API with the same amount of filler and thoroughly mixing them together using a mortar and pestle. Once thoroughly mixed, add more filler in an equivalent amount to the powder in the mortar and repeat the process of geometric dilution. To ensure thorough mixing, a tracer such as colored powder can be added to the mixture. Using a tracer is recommended as it is difficult to visually inspect and assess the homogeneity of the mixture when the powders are all the same color (e.g. white). In the case that the color of the powder is not distributed evenly following geometric dilution, the process needs to be reviewed by the compounder and the powder needs additional mixing. Geometric dilution will be discussed in more detail in Chapter 6. Some APIs may not be available in micronized form – reduced particle size – and will require trituration alone before adding the filler.

Trituration is the application of adequate force against the bottom and sides of the mortar. This is best achieved by using the pestle to apply pressure in circular motions and moving in both clockwise and counterclockwise directions. Prior to trituration, ensure that the mortar is firmly grasped and avoid providing too much force with the pestle or the mortar can shatter. After the trituration of any powder, utilize a rubber spatula and remove any powder that is stuck on the sides of the mortar. Trituration will be discussed in more detail in Chapter 6.

The physical process of compounding capsules will differ depending on if they are being hand-packed (the punch method) or prepared using a capsule machine. Capsule machines are available in 100 count and 300 count quantities for varying capsule sizes, and the process for how to use them can differ slightly depending on the manufacturer. The standard capsule size is #3. The lower the number, the larger the size of the capsule will be. Some medications can be compounded using a #4 capsule, which may be more beneficial for smaller patients such as cats. When using a capsule machine, the compounder should avoid pouring the entire quantity of powder on the machine at once as well as avoiding adding the powder directly to the center each time. Both of these processes can lead to overweight capsules in the middle and underweight capsules around the edges.

The hand-packed process follows the same steps as above for combining powders using geometric dilution. The proper procedure differs once the powders are appropriately combined. The powder mixture will be placed on powder paper, an ointment slab, or in a weigh boat. The mixture should be smoothed out with a height approximately the same length as half of the capsule body. Once the two pieces of the capsule (head and body) are separated, the body of the capsule is repeatedly punched into the powder until full. Some compounders find it easiest to use a twisting motion while punching the capsule body into the powder. Either technique is acceptable as long as one is selected and used every time. The head of the capsule will then be reconnected to the body, and each capsule should be weighed to confirm that the amount of powder added is within the appropriate range. Once the correct weight is verified, the head of the capsule should be locked into the body, and any powder residue wiped off with a lint-free cloth or paper towel. The appropriate range can be determined with the following formula:

$$\frac{\text{Total weight (grams)}}{100} = \text{grams / capsule target weight.}$$

The target weight should be recorded as well as both the highest and lowest weights from the capsules that are weighed out. Divide the highest weight by the target weight and record the answer as a percentage. Then, divide the lowest weight by the target weight and record the answer as a percentage. The range should be within 95–105%, which allows for a ±5% error.

For capsules that contain beads, no packing statistics need to be completed. The individual capsule should be opened, and the contents placed into a weigh boat. The contents can then be split into halves, thirds, or fourths depending on the desired strength. In the case that the practice has omeprazole 20-mg capsules, but a patient requires 5 mg of omeprazole per dose, the compounder would split the contents of the original manufactured capsule into four equal amounts and then pour each amount into its own capsules, creating four compounded capsules with a strength of 5 mg. The capsules that are being used for the compound can be held in gloved hands or in a capsule machine. Some compounders purchase specific tools to transfer the beads with such as a small funnel or scoop, while others create their own funnel using paper or simply pour the beads from the weigh boat into the new capsule.

Compounding Formulations to Avoid

Compounded medications do not always reach appropriate therapeutic concentrations or maintain their stability as expected, and some compounds require advanced procedures to ensure that they are formulated well and will maintain their stability. One example of the importance of using the appropriate ingredients when compounding medications is with compounded omeprazole liquid suspension. The rate of degradation of omeprazole increases as the pH becomes more acidic as the drug is a lipophilic weak base [23]. In the USP Compounding Compendium formulation, sodium bicarbonate is utilized to maintain the pH of the compound in an aqueous vehicle.

As discussed in Chapter 2, published studies have been completed that prove that many compounded products are not bioequivalent with FDA-approved products. Studies also indicate that medications compounded for transdermal use may not be bioavailable at all and, therefore, should not be prescribed using this route of administration. Many of these studies are discussed in previous chapters. The compounder can find studies where compounded products failed by completing proper research, but there are products that the authors recommend not compounding in-house and instead outsourcing to a reliable compounding pharmacy. These products include sterile products (injectable and ophthalmic), chemotherapy medications and other hazardous medications included on the NIOSH list, and any compounds that require bulk powder that is not USP grade. More information regarding finding a quality compounding pharmacy can be found in Chapter 4.

Formulation Development Process

The process for developing a new compounding formulation varies depending on the availability of a formula in the Compounding Compendium or from another reputable source, if stability-indicating assays are available, and if USP default dating is appropriate for the patient's treatment period. In the case that a recipe is already available, the compounder first needs to check that the recipe is complete, calculations are done appropriately, all ingredients are USP grade, and a stability-indicating assay has been completed. Once the recipe is reviewed and considered to be acceptable, an MFR and compounding record (CR) must be developed. Following the development of the appropriate documentation, a test product should be compounded. Testing the formula allows the compounder to adjust any steps in the process, if necessary, determine what each ingredient looks like so appropriate information can be added to the MFR, and confirm that the final product looks as expected. The required components of the MFR and CR are listed below in Table 5.10, and more information can be found in Chapter 6.

When a formulation cannot be found in the USP Compounding Compendium and another source has to be used, the study should be reviewed in-depth, and references pulled to confirm that a stability-indicating assay has been done. Refer to Chapter 3 for additional discussion about this. Upon the verification of a stability-indicating assay, the appropriate documentation must be created and a test product compounded.

If no formulations can be found, then the process must be started from scratch. Formulations for similar products can be evaluated to provide a starting place for the new compounding formula. The active ingredient must be thoroughly researched including its solubility, lipophilicity/hydrophilicity, chemical grade from available suppliers, and the need for excipients. The calculations will reflect the desired strength and include any necessary excipients in appropriate quantities. The MFR and CR can then be created, including a BUD that reflects the amount of water present in the compound and how it is administered using USP default dating. The formulation needs to be tested, and if the compounder is interested in extending the BUD, a baseline assay should be completed. Figure 5.11 shows a flowchart of the formulation development process.

Table 5.10 Comparison of MFR and CR.

Master formulation record	Compounding record
Name, strength or activity, and dosage form of the CNSP	Name, strength or activity, and dosage form of the CNSP
Identities and amounts of all components; if applicable, relevant characteristics of components (e.g. particle size, salt form, purity grade, solubility)	Date – or date and time – of preparation of the CNSP
Container closure system(s)	Assigned internal identification number (e.g. prescription, order, or lot number)
Complete instructions for preparing the CNSP including equipment, supplies, and description of compounding steps	A method to identify the individuals involved in the compounding process and individuals verifying the final CNSP
Physical description of the final CNSP	Name, vendor or manufacturer, lot number, and expiration date of each component
BUD and storage requirements	Weight or measurement of each component
Reference source to support the assigned BUD	Total quantity of the CNSP compounded
If applicable, calculations to determine and verify quantities and/or concentrations of components and strength or activity of the API(s)	Assigned BUD and storage requirements
Labeling requirements (e.g. shake well)	If applicable, calculations to determine and verify quantities and/or concentrations of components and strength or activity of the API(s)
Quality control (QC) procedures (e.g. pH testing, visual inspection) and expected results	Physical description of the final CNSP
Other information needed to describe the compounding process and ensure repeatability (e.g. adjusting pH, temperature)	Results of quality control procedures (e.g. pH testing and visual inspection)
	MFR reference for the CNSP

Boxes in green are the identical for both documents. *Source:* Adapted from USP (2022).

Developing a Compounding Formula: Example 1 (USP Compounding Compendium)

A veterinarian at your practice is interested in compounding a gabapentin liquid product that does not require refrigeration to make it easier to administered doses to large patients and prevent clients from accidentally leaving the product out of the refrigerator. As the "responsible person" (defined in Chapter 6), you agree that a compounded formulation would be beneficial and begin the process of developing a compounding formula. Knowing that USP has a Compounding Compendium with accurate formulations, you start your search there.

You find that there is a gabapentin compounded oral suspension formulation that does not require storage at refrigerated temperatures, which is exactly what you are looking for. You review the formulation and determine that the compounding process is feasible with your nonsterile compounding equipment, a stability-indicating assay was completed, and the BUD is not more than 90 days after the date compounded. In order to determine the concentration for the formula, you

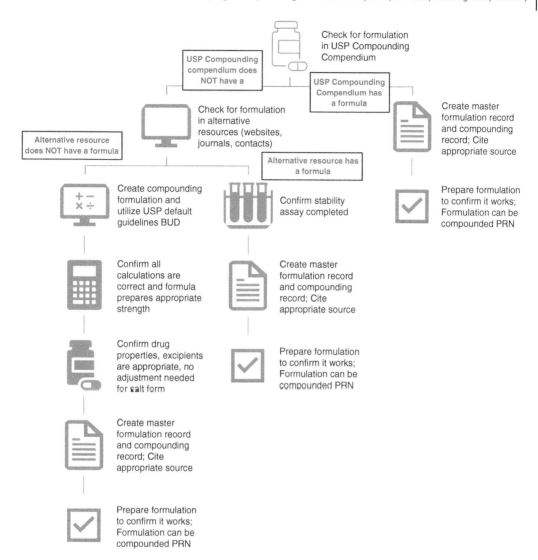

Figure 5.11 Steps to developing a compounding formulation.

must divide the amount of powder (in milligrams) that is supposed to be dissolved in the liquid vehicle (ml). The formulation states to dissolve 15 g of gabapentin in 150 ml of the oral mix vehicle

$$\frac{15000\,\text{mg}}{150\,\text{mL}} = 100\,\text{mg}\,/\,\text{mL}.$$

The concentration for the formula is 100 mg/ml. This product contains twice the amount of mg/ml as the manufactured gabapentin oral solution (50 mg/ml). Next you need to confirm that you have access to the ingredients as USP grade if they are not available as a manufactured product. The formulation says you are able to use gabapentin 300-mg capsules (Apotex brand) or gabapentin powder. If you have access to that brand of manufactured capsules, legally they should be utilized. If you are unable to order this brand of gabapentin, then you will start looking at compounding wholesalers for the appropriate grade of bulk powder. Unfortunately, your veterinary suppliers do not carry this brand of gabapentin capsules. You do, however, find that the USP-grade bulk powder is available from all of the compounding wholesalers you use. Oral mix, a combination or suspending and sweetening agent, is available from the noted company.

Knowing your concentration of the compounded suspension and your ingredients, you can now create the MFR and CR. Since both documents have similar requirements, your practice has determined in your SOP that it is easier to include all of the pertinent information on one form. The document is kept electronically on all of the computers and printed out for patient specific compounding. You create a new formulation online and input the name and strength of the product ("Gabapentin 100-mg/ml Oral Compounded Suspension"), the BUD ("90 days"), storage requirements ("Room Temperature"), copy the procedure for how to compound the medication from the Compounding Compendium, and create space to complete the calculations necessary if a client requires less than or more than 150 ml.

When your ingredients arrive, you will add in their NDC, Lot #, manufacturer, and expiration date in the unfortunate event that a product would get recalled. On your document, you also include that your reference is the USP Compounding Compendium and that the following auxiliary labels/statements must be added – shake well, notation that it is a compounded product, and expiration date where you will write in the patient/product specific BUD. The practice has developed a quality assurance/quality control check list and you pull this from the SOP and utilize it for every compound.

Once your document is complete and contains all of the requirements for an MFR and CR, you have a coworker double check the calculations to confirm the strength of the product and ensure if a different quantity will be prepared that the formulas placed in the document are correct. After receiving confirmation that everything is accurate, you will create a test batch of the product. Testing a compounded preparation confirms what the final product should look like and that the drug suspends appropriately in the vehicle. This also serves as a verification that your compounding steps are written accurately.

When you feel comfortable with the product (after confirming it suspends properly), the formulation can be prepared for individual patients as needed. A sample compounding sheet that includes the requirements for both the MFR and CR can be found in Chapter 6.

Developing a Compounding Formula: Example 2 (Stability-Indicating Assay)

A technician at your practice wants to discuss the possibility of preparing an enalapril compounded oral suspension that has a concentration of less than 10 mg/ml for use in smaller patients. You currently compound the 10-mg/ml concentration, which is a formulation from the USP Compounding Compendium, but you agree that a lower concentration would be very beneficial for your smaller patients as well as "pocket pets." As the "responsible person" (defined in Chapter 6), you begin the process of developing a compounding formula. You already prepare the formula in the USP Compounding Compendium and, therefore, must consider other places to look for a formulation. Some of your compounding wholesalers provide consultation services, but they charge a fee, so you reserve that as a last resort option. The "Compounding Today" website shows there is a compounded formula, but you are not a member and do not plan on paying for the membership at this time. You remember though that you have a membership to the "IJPC" and search the journal website for formulas.

You find a formula for enalapril 1-mg/ml compounded oral suspension. This strength of enalapril will make it far easier to dose your small patients. First you want to confirm that this is a stability-indicating study. You look under the heading "Stability" and find a cited study – *Stability of Extemporaneously Prepared Enalapril Maleate Suspensions in Glass Bottles and Plastic Syringes*. You must now review the study and you remember from Chapter 3 that the key words you are looking for are *stability-indicating* and *forced degradation*. The study discusses the forced degradation experiments that occurred where the compounded suspensions were subjected to high heat. Now that you have confirmed the study is stability indicating, you review the formula verifying that the compounding process is feasible with your nonsterile compounding equipment and determine that the BUD is not more than 91 days after the date compounded at either room temperature or refrigerated temperature. You confirm that this information was pulled from the cited study appropriately and see that the study notes that the BUD is not more than 90 days at room temperature or refrigerated temperature as the study did not pull concentrations after 90 days. Therefore, your BUD will not be more than 90 days at room temperature.

In order to confirm that the concentration for the formula is correct, you must divide the amount of powder (in milligrams) that is supposed to be dissolved by the liquid vehicle (ml). The formulation states to dissolve 10 10-mg tablets of enalapril in 100 ml of (1 : 1) Ora-Plus: Ora-Sweet

$$10\,mg \times 10\,(tables) = 100\,mg\,\frac{100\,mg}{100\,mL} = 1\,mg\,/\,mL.$$

The concentration for the formula is confirmed to be 1 mg/ml. You also remember that Chapter 3 mentions that the USP allows for the bracketing of concentrations. Since there are stability data for enalapril 1-mg/ml compounded oral suspension AND enalapril 10-mg/ml compounded oral suspension and they use the same formulation, you can technically compound any of the strengths in between. However, you determine that a concentration of 1 mg/ml works the best for your practice.

Next you need to confirm that you have access to the ingredients as USP grade if they are not available as a manufactured product. The formulation utilized enalapril 10-mg tablets (Vasotec brand). You are able to order that exact product from one of your veterinary wholesalers and you already stock Ora-Plus and Ora-Sweet as you use them for other formulations you compound.

Knowing your concentration of the compounded suspension and your ingredients, you can now create the MFR and CR. Since both documents have similar requirements, your practice has determined in your SOP that it is easier to include all of the pertinent information on one form. The document is kept electronically on all of the computers and printed out for patient specific compounding. You create a new formulation online and input the name and strength of the product ("Enalapril 1-mg/ml Oral Compounded Suspension"), the BUD ("90 days"), storage requirements ("Room Temperature"), copy the procedure for how to compound the medication from the formula published by IJPC under "Method of Preparation," and create space to complete the calculations necessary if a client requires less than or more than 100 ml.

When your tablets arrive, you will add in their NDC, Lot #, manufacturer, and expiration date in the unfortunate event that they would get recalled. You also add in the same information for both the Ora-Sweet and Ora-Plus products. On your document, you include the citation for the IJPC study for your reference and that the following auxiliary labels/statements must be added – shake well, notation that it is a compounded product, and expiration date where you will write in the patient/product specific BUD. The practice has developed a quality assurance/quality control check list and you pull this from the SOP and utilize it for every compound.

Once your document is complete and contains all of the requirements for an MFR and CR, you have a coworker double check the calculations to confirm the strength of the product and ensure if a different quantity will be prepared that the formulas placed in the document are correct. After receiving confirmation that everything is accurate you will create a test batch of the product. Testing a compounded preparation confirms what the final product should look like and that the drug suspends appropriately in the vehicle.

When you feel comfortable with the product (after confirming it suspends properly), the formulation can be prepared for individual patients as needed. A sample compounding sheet that includes the requirements for both the MFR and CR can be found in Chapter 6.

Several months after you develop this formulation, you see that the USP has added a monograph for enalapril 1-mg/ml suspension (nonveterinary). You review this monograph and are happy to see that the formulation and BUD align with the one you developed. You then add the USP monograph as a second reference on your MFR document.

Compounding Formulation Assessment

To summarize important aspects of this chapter, there are five main questions to consider during formulation development prior to the addition of any new compound to a formulary. If you cannot answer them all, then more research should be completed prior to the development of the compound. These questions are:

1) What are the properties of the API and excipients and are there any potential interactions that have been reported?
2) Do the ingredients meet the chemical grade standards put forth by the USP?
3) Will the dosage form selected allow for adequate absorption of the drug while avoiding potential adverse effects?
4) Is the BUD that is assigned appropriate (e.g. USP Compounding Compendium monograph, USP guidelines for default dating, and study with stability-indicating assay)?
5) Does the disease state I am treating have a discernible effect that can be monitored or how will it be determined that the compounded product is effective?

Sources that were referred to throughout the text can be found in Table 5.11.

Table 5.11 Sources referenced in text.

Reference name	Website	Provided information	Membership required?
Ingredient selection			
Guidance for industry: ICHQ7 Good Manufacturing Guidance for Active Pharmaceuticals	https://www.fda.gov/drugs/guidance-compliance-regulatory-information/guidances-drugs	Provides guidance for good manufacturing practices (GMP) for the manufacturing of APIs	No
Solubility			
National Library of Medicine (NLM) PubChem	https://pubchem.ncbi.nlm.nih.gov	Provides summary of chemical characteristics of drugs	No

Table 5.11 (Continued)

Reference name	Website	Provided information	Membership required?
	Partition coefficient		
DrugBank Online	https://go.drugbank.com	Provides access to API pharmaceutical properties	No
	Hazardous drugs		
NIOSH List of Antineoplastics and Other Hazardous Drugs in Healthcare Settings	https://www.cdc.gov/niosh/docs/2016-161/default.html	Provides a list of hazardous drugs and their American Hospital Formulary Service (AHFS) classification	No
	Formulation resources		
USP Compounding Compendium	https://www.usp.org/products/usp-compounding-compendium	Provides access to compounding studies and literature; Only formulation resource guaranteed to have stability-indicating data	Yes
NLM PubMed	https://pubmed.ncbi.nlm.nih.gov	Provides access to citations to biomedical literature	No
IJPC	https://ijpc.com	Provides access to compounding studies and literature	Yes
Trissel's Stability of Compounding Formulations	(Textbook only)	Provides access to compounding studies	No but textbook must be purchased
Compounding Today	https://compoundingtoday.com	Provides access to compounding studies and literature	Yes

References

1 (1994). ASHP technical assistance bulletin on compounding nonsterile products in pharmacies. American Society of Hospital Pharmacists. *Am. J. Hosp. Pharm.* 51 (11): 1441–1448. PMID: 7942879.

2 German, A.J., Cannon, M.J., Dye, C. et al. (2005). Oesophageal strictures in cats associated with doxycycline therapy. *J. Feline Med. Surg.* 7 (1): 33–41. https://doi.org/10.1016/j.jfms.2004.04.001. PMID: 15686972.

3 Colucci, G., Santamaria-Echart, A., Silva, S.C. et al. (2020). Development of water-in-oil emulsions as delivery vehicles and testing with a natural antimicrobial extract. *Molecules* 25 (9): 2105. https://doi.org/10.3390/molecules25092105. PMID: 32365923; PMCID: PMC7248747.

4 Paudel, K.S., Milewski, M., Swadley, C.L. et al. (2010). Challenges and opportunities in dermal/transdermal delivery. *Ther. Deliv.* 1 (1): 109–131. https://doi.org/10.4155/tde.10.16. PMID: 21132122; PMCID: PMC2995530.

5 Purnamawati, S., Indrastuti, N., Danarti, R., and Saefudin, T. (2017). The role of moisturizers in addressing various kinds of dermatitis: a review. *Clin. Med. Res.* 15 (3–4): 75–87. https://doi.org/10.3121/cmr.2017.1363. Epub 2017 Dec 11. PMID: 29229630; PMCID: PMC5849435.

6 Cohn, J.A., Brown, E.T., Reynolds, W.S. et al. (2016). An update on the use of transdermal oxybutynin in the management of overactive bladder disorder. *Ther. Adv. Urol.* 8 (2): 83–90. https://doi.org/10.1177/1756287215626312.

7 Gavazzoni Dias, M.F. (2015). Hair cosmetics: an overview. *Int. J. Trichol.* 7 (1): 2–15. https://doi.org/10.4103/0974-7753.153450. PMID: 25878443; PMCID: PMC4387693.

8 Gennari, C.G.M., Selmin, F., Minghetti, P., and Cilurzo, F. (2019). Medicated foams and film forming dosage forms as tools to improve the thermodynamic activity of drugs to be administered through the skin. *Curr. Drug Deliv.* 16 (5): 461–471. https://doi.org/10.2174/1567201816666190118124439. PMID: 30657040; PMCID: PMC6637090.

9 Hua, S. (2019). Physiological and pharmaceutical considerations for rectal drug formulations. *Front. Pharmacol.* 10: 1196. https://doi.org/10.3389/fphar.2019.01196. PMID: 31680970; PMCID: PMC6805701.

10 USP (2019). *USP General Chapter <795> Pharmaceutical Compounding – Nonsterile Preparations.*

11 *ACS reagent chemicals.* ACS Publications, American Chemical Society. https://pubs.acs.org/isbn/9780841230460 (accessed 24 March 2023).

12 CFR – Code of Federal Regulations Title 21. data.fda.gov https://www.accessdata.fda.gov/scripts/cdrh/cfdocs/cfcfr/CFRSearch.cfm?fr=216.23 (accessed 24 March 2023).

13 Savjani, K.T., Gajjar, A.K., and Savjani, J.K. (2012). Drug solubility: importance and enhancement techniques. *ISRN Pharm.* 2012: 195727. https://doi.org/10.5402/2012/195727. Epub 2012 Jul 5. PMID: 22830056; PMCID: PMC3399483.

14 Bannan, C.C., Calabró, G., Kyu, D.Y., and Mobley, D.L. (2016). Calculating partition coefficients of small molecules in octanol/water and cyclohexane/water. *J. Chem. Theory Comput.* 12 (8): 4015–4024. https://doi.org/10.1021/acs.jctc.6b00449. Epub 2016 Aug 1. PMID: 27434695; PMCID: PMC5053177.

15 Tsantili-Kakoulidou, A. and Demopoulos, V.J. (2021). Drug-like properties and fraction lipophilicity index as a combined metric. *ADMET DMPK* 9 (3): 177–190. https://doi.org/10.5599/admet.1022. PMID: 35300360; PMCID: PMC8920096.

16 Ditzinger, F., Price, D.J., Ilie, A.R. et al. (2019). Lipophilicity and hydrophobicity considerations in bio-enabling oral formulations approaches – a PEARRL review. *J. Pharm. Pharmacol.* 71 (4): 464–482. https://doi.org/10.1111/jphp.12984. Epub 2018 Aug 2. PMID: 30070363.

17 Vázquez-Blanco, S., González-Freire, L., Dávila-Pousa, M.C., and Crespo-Diz, C. (2018). pH determination as a quality standard for the elaboration of oral liquid compounding formula. *Farm. Hosp.* 42 (6): 221–227. English. https://doi.org/10.7399/fh.10932. PMID: 30381041.

18 Gabrič, A., Hodnik, Ž., and Pajk, S. (2022). Oxidation of drugs during drug product development: problems and solutions. *Pharmaceutics* 14 (2): 325. https://doi.org/10.3390/pharmaceutics14020325. PMID: 35214057; PMCID: PMC8876153.

19 (2021). Identifying color additives in regulated drug products. Institute For Safe Medication Practices. https://www.ismp.org/resources/identifying-color-additives-regulated-drug-products (accessed 18 June 2021).

20 Paulekuhn, G.S., Dressman, J.B., and Saal, C. (2007). Trends in active pharmaceutical ingredient salt selection based on analysis of the orange book database. *J. Med. Chem.* 50: 6665–6672. https://doi.org/10.1021/jm701032y.

21 (2016). Antineoplastic & other hazardous drugs in healthcare (2016). Centers for Disease Control and Prevention. https://www.cdc.gov/niosh/docs/2016-161/default.html (accessed 31 March 2017).

22 Compounded Preparation Monographs (CPM). USP https://www.usp.org/compounding/compounded-preparation-monographs (accessed 24 March 2023).

23 Bestebreurtje, P., Roeleveld, N., Knibbe, C.A.J. et al. (2020). Development and stability study of an omeprazole suppository for infants. *Eur. J. Drug Metab. Pharmacokinet.* 45: 627–633. https://doi.org/10.1007/s13318-020-00629-1.

6

Compounding in House

Documentation

Chapter 5 briefly covered the requirement for the documentation of compounded medications. The formulas being utilized must be easily replicated, and the master formulation record (MFR) and compounding record (CR) must be accessible in written form or electronically. Compounds that are dispensed must comply with any applicable state and federal laws and regulations, including storing records for required periods of time. For additional information on laws and regulations for compounding, refer to Chapter 1. Records for individual patient compounds must include a copy of the prescription, MFR, and CR. The MFR and CR can be combined into a single document as long as all of the requirements for each are met, or they can be developed as two separate documents.

Master Formulation Record

An MFR includes all necessary information relating to the formula and appropriate procedures that must be followed in order to safely compound the product. These records are required for any medications that are compounded in batches or are compounded more than one time. An MFR is usually developed by the "responsible person" and should be reviewed and updated regularly. The "responsible person" or "designated person" is the individual assigned to be accountable and responsible for compounding operations and performance. They oversee both the facility and the personnel. If the responsibilities are too much for one individual to handle, then more than one person can be designated. It outlines how to compound the medication, what ingredients are utilized, and the resource that provided the beyond-use date (BUD) and/or where the formula reference is located.

Compounding Record

A CR is created every time a formula is compounded per an individual patient prescription. The CR contains the specific information for the prescription that was compounded on a specific day including that individual prescription's quantity, assigned BUD, date of compounding, and the person who compounded it as well as who approved it. The information related to the ingredient's sources (Manufacturer and National Drug Codes – NDCs), lot numbers, and expiry dates are also recorded here. The inclusion of the drug information should **never** be skipped because if an active

Drug Compounding for Veterinary Professionals, First Edition. Lauren R. Eichstadt Forsythe and Alexandria E. Gochenauer.
© 2023 John Wiley & Sons, Inc. Published 2023 by John Wiley & Sons, Inc.
Companion Website: www.wiley.com/go/forsythe/drug

pharmaceutical ingredient (API) or excipient is recalled, this is the only way the compounder is able to determine which patients received the recalled product.

The MFR and CR do have several requirements in common that makes it very easy to combine the two documents into one all-inclusive document. The requirements for each document and the notation of which requirements are similar between the two can be found in Chapter 5 (see Table 5.10). An example document containing the requirements for both the MFR and CR (see Figure 6.1) and a completed example (see Figure 6.2) can be found below.

Formulation Record Components

The MFR and CR, or combined document, must be filled out in its entirety. The name of the compounded product, concentration, and dosage form will be provided by the monograph that is followed or the resource used to develop the formulation. This confirms that the compounder is preparing the appropriate compound. Any time the formulation is adjusted, the protocol number or version, effective date, and documentation of who developed and verified it must be updated, which allows those preparing compounds to confirm that they are following the most up-to-date version of the formulation. The inclusion of who developed and verified the formulation provides the information of the person who can answer any questions that may arise. The date of when the compound was prepared supplies a method to easily find that the completed documentation to corroborate the compound was made to the appropriate specifications.

A benefit to combining the MFR and CR is that if anticipatory compounding is completed, the prescription label can be considered the CR. However, this is only true if the prescription label that is generated includes the lot number and expiration date for each compound dispensed out of the batch.

The lot number is an internal designation describing when the compounded preparation was made and whether it was the first compound prepared on that day, the second compound, the third compound, and so on. Using this process does require a written standard operating procedure (SOP) documenting how this is appropriately completed. An example of creating a lot number is shown below.

The date today is June 1, 2023, and the veterinarian has been very busy, already having prepared four compounds. A patient has difficulty swallowing capsules and tablets, so the client has asked about the possibility of giving the patient the medication as a liquid. You already have a formulation for this product as a liquid and head to the compounding room to prepare it. The way your internal lot numbers are assigned is based on the date. A whiteboard in the compounding room documents the last compound prepared was number 4.

The format for your lot number(s) is: Today's date (XX/XX/XX) + The number of the compound to be completed (XX). In this example, today's date is 06/01/23 and this is the fifth (05) compound to be prepared. Therefore, you write the lot number on the compounding form as 06012305.

Another important part of the documentation is the total quantity that is being compounded for the patient. The quantity is required in order to complete the appropriate calculations for all of the ingredients that are used.

The section "Quality Assurance and Quality Control" of the document is the ingredients for the formula. These ingredients, as discussed in Chapter 5, should be listed with the full drug name, drug strength if a manufactured product, a physical description, quantity needed (after completing the calculations), and the supplied lot #, expiration date, manufacturer, and NDC of the product.

Any calculations that need to be completed are listed in the calculations and measurements section. Equations can be preprepared as in Figure 6.2, where the compounder only has to write

Name of compounded product:	Protocol number / version:	
Concentration:	Effective date:	
Dosage form:	Developed by:	
Route of administration:	Verified by:	
Date of Preparation:	*Internal Lot # :*	
	Quantity being compounded:	

Formula

Ingredients:	Quantities:	Product description:	Lot #, Expiration Date, Manufacturer, NDC:
_____	_____	_____	_____
_____	_____	_____	_____
_____	_____	_____	_____

Prepared by: _____   *Checked by*: _____

Additional information about ingredients:

Calculations and measurements:

Ingredient 1 _____ calculated weight = _____ actual weight = _____
Ingredient 2 _____ calculated weight = _____ actual weight = _____
Ingredient 3 _____ calculated weight = _____ actual weight = _____

Required equipment / instruments / materials:

Process for compounding:

Step 1 _____
Step 2 _____
Step 3 _____

Quality controls:

Final product should be _____ *in color, (cloudy / clear), and have no phase separation present.*

QC testing required (circle)?   pH   Bubble Test   Other _____
QC testing passed (check)?   □ Yes □ No   □ Yes □ No   □ Yes □ No
Verified by ; _____

Packaging (container system):

Stability and storage:
Beyond use date per monograph: _____
Beyond usedate ofpatient specificproduct: _____
Store at (room temperature / refrigerated temperature / frozen)

Labeling:

[prescription label for patient attached here]

Required auxiliary labels:

Training required: □ Yes _____   □ No

References / resources:

Figure 6.1   Combined MFR/CR document example. Information with white background is required by the MFR; information with yellow background is required by the CR; information with green background is required by *both* MFR and CR.

in the quantity to be dispensed to complete calculations or the compounding instructions can be written to provide information to complete the calculations. The authors recommend that the equations are preprepared to prevent calculation errors. If any products are weighed out, the actual weight reading from the scale should be written or printed out on receipt paper and taped to the actual weight portion of this section. Once this information is recorded and the

Oral Liquid Compounding Sheet

Product: __ABC Drug Suspension 10 mg/mL__   BUD: **30 days**   Qty: __30__ mL

5mL Minimum
5mL Increments

Date: __6__ / __1__ / __23__   Lot: __06012301__   Exp: __7__ / __1__ / __23__

Product/Ingredients			Quantity
ABC Drug Tablets	NDC: __12345 - 678 - 10__		__6 tablets__
Lot: __45678__ Exp: __10/2023__	Mfr: __ABC Drug Manufacturer__		
Bitterness Suppressor			__0.3 gm__
Lot: __187033/B__ Exp: __4/2024__	Mfr: __Medisca__		
Syrpalta	NDC: __0395 - 2661 - 16__		QS to __30__ mL
Lot: __A73314__ Exp: __6/2025__	Mfr: Humco		
ABC Drug Tablets	$\dfrac{10\,mg/mL\ (\,Total\,)\ mL}{50mg\ tabs}$ = ABC Drug Tablets	10 mg/mL (__30__ mL) ÷ 50 mg tabs = __6__ tabs	
Bitterness Suppressor	0.01 x (Total) gm = Bitterness Suppressor gm	0.01 x __30__ = __0.3__ gm	
Syrpalta	Syrpalta mL = QS to (Total mL)	Q.S. to __30__ mL	

Optional flavor Powder/Liquid (please record flavor): __None__			__None__
Lot: Exp: Mfr:	0.03 x	mL = _____ g or mL	

Directions:
- Calculate ingredient amounts using the equations above, please show your work.
- Assemble and dispense the ingredients, fill in the lot numbers, and ask for a pharmacist check.
- Place the tablets in a mortar and triturate into a fine powder.
    - If adding flavor powder or bitterness suppressor, add and triturate with drug powder.
    - If adding liquid flavor or bitterness suppressor, add to vial after Syrpalta.
- Add a small amount of Syrpalta to the powder and mix into a smooth paste.
- Add enough Syrpalta to make the paste into a liquid and transfer to an oral dispensing vial.
- Add Syrpalta to the mortar and scrape all residue with a rubber spatula into the vial.
- Add Syrpalta to final volume in the vial.
- Label with
    - Shake Well/Refrigerate
    - Expiration Date
    - Compounded Drug
- Affix a patient label to the back of this sheet.
- BUD 30 days

Prepared By: __PI__

Checked By: __TI__

Place patient label here

Figure 6.2   Completed MFR/CR.

Accuracy Check and Physical Quality Assessment:
- Correct formulation has been prepared (check against original order)
- Correct ingredients (identities, purities, and amounts) have been used
- Appropriate beyond use date has been assigned
- No evidence of particulates or other foreign matter
- No evidence of other apparent visual defect
- Label information verified for accuracy
- Container-closure checked for integrity (i.e. no leaks, cracks)
- Color of preparation: ___purple___
- Final volume of preparation (for solutions, suspension, etc) ___30 ml___

Characteristics	Expected	Actual (circle one)
Uniformity	Uniform	(Uniform) Not uniform
Clarity	Cloudy	Clear (Cloudy)
Coalescence/Phase separation	Not present	Present (Not present)

This formulation has met QA standards documented above:

☒ Yes

☐ No (document remedial action taken in the Pharmacy Notes section below)

Checking PharmD/CPhT initial ___TI___

Ref: REFERENCE ADDED HERE

General Handling Precautions
N/A

Spill Management
N/A

Reason for use of bulk powder
N/A

Remedial Action Taken
None

Figure 6.2 (Continued)

calculations for product quantities are complete and drawn up or weighed out, the formula should be checked by a second person.

Required equipment, instruments, and materials must be included in the document. There is a slew of glassware that can be used and a variety of sizes for each glassware type. Stating the exact type of glassware used including the size increases the quality of the compound being prepared. The process for compounding is another document requirement and must detail each individual step that is completed during the preparation. On the off chance that the staff member who typically compounds medication is not available, another person must be able to review the compounding steps and be able to prepare the compound without confusion. Within the compounding process, the details of what equipment to use and when to use it should be covered as well as the dispensing container, labeling, and any additional requirements.

Other information that is typically pulled from the monograph and must be included is the packaging or container system being used for dispensation, expected stability, and storage of the product. This includes the standard BUD and product-specific BUD based on the date the compound is prepared, the patient specific prescription label, and any required auxiliary labels. Auxiliary labels highlight the significance of storage or product requirements such as "shake well," "keep refrigerated," and "expiration date: _____." It must be designated on the label of the official compounded veterinary preparation that it is "compounded," and the word "veterinary" must follow the official name (e.g. Enalapril Compounded Oral Suspension, and Veterinary).

In the case that special training is required prior to preparing the compound, this should also be documented and described. One example of additional training is if a compound must be a certain pH in order to maintain stability. The compounder will need to know how to utilize either pH test strips or a pH meter. The final requirement of the document is the references and/or resources used to prepare the formulation. The United States Pharmacopeia (USP) Compounding Compendium and other references may change over time, and noting the resource used helps the compounder confirm that they are using the most up-to-date and accurate formulation.

The importance of quality assurance (QA) and quality control (QC) is discussed more in depth in the following section. However, the specific items to be evaluated for the formulation should be included on the CR to ensure that all the important aspects are verified and document this verification. The documentation must have a way to verify the quality of product(s) being prepared and dispensed as a final verification. See Figure 6.2 for an example of a completed document that includes the MFR and CR.

Quality Assurance and Quality Control

QA and QC are extremely important to maintaining the quality of compounded products. QA is the system put in place by the practice of steps taken to ensure that proper standards are being upheld. This is what provides a client the confidence that quality conditions are being achieved. QC is the actual process of inspection and verification or other activities that are used to satisfy requirements for quality. This is the process of focusing on meeting expectations of quality products. Another way to compare the two concepts is that QA is a prevention strategy, whereas QC is a method of detection. Examples of QA methods are monitoring the potency, sterility, and stability of a compound such as with a yearly stability indicating assay spot check, confirming the certificate of analysis (CoA) of products received quarterly, biannual review of compounding formulations, and completing a random sterility test on a product approaching its expiration date. Random sterility testing would be very easy to do if the clinic prepares anticipatory products, but a practice batch can also be prepared by those involved in compounding to facilitate this process. Examples of QC are focused on daily operations including physically observing a final product to verify it looks like it is supposed to, confirming that appropriate container closure systems are used for dispensed products including a push-in seal and syringes for oral products, and validating that all sections on the documentation are filled out for a compounded preparation. The items included in QC are typically those that are checked prior to dispensing the final product such as shown in Figure 6.2.

There are QC measures that are obvious in nature, but there are also some that may not be immediately recognized. USP 795 and 797 address the quality of nonsterile and sterile compounded preparations, respectively. Veterinarians who compound medications should verify that they have a program or strategy in place to ensure the quality all the medications they compound. This can include the verification of compounding ingredients and quantities at multiple steps throughout the compounding process and descriptions of each ingredient being used as well as expected characteristics of the product in the MFR. Each ingredient that is utilized by the compounder must have a CoA and material safety data sheet that are easily accessible. These documents should be reviewed by the compounder any time an ingredient is ordered and received by the practice as an additional QA measure.

In order to guarantee the quality of the compounds being prepared, the owner of the practice needs to take personal responsibility or delegate the responsibility to another member of the practice. The person(s) is then responsible for ensuring that the appropriate laws and regulations are followed, compounding practices are done appropriately, and that anyone who may compound is properly trained in QA and QC. The standards at any practice start at the top and trickle down eventually leading to a change in culture. Without execution by the leader or director, QC standards will not gain traction. Effectively implementing a process of QA requires processes that make it clear what is expected (e.g. a double check at certain points) and make it easier to do the correct versus incorrect action (e.g. organization of compounding ingredients to decrease the likelihood of grabbing the wrong ingredient). Having a single person with "ownership" of this process will be more effective than general education and reminders.

The previous chapters in this text have mentioned that the rules and regulations surrounding compounding are constantly evolving. The development of new and interesting dosage forms, improved delivery systems, and additional or reviewed guidance from the Food and Drug Administration (FDA) and USP allow compounders to develop and refine their craft. Properly educating staff and staying up to date with continuing education is crucial to the quality of compounded medications. There is no part of healthcare that is static, including veterinary medicine. We must always remind ourselves and those around us that we cannot abstain from learning what is new, and it is our responsibility to pass correct information on to our colleagues and peers that can benefit from our knowledge.

The overall goal of QA and QC in the compounding process is to reduce variance and prevent mistakes. A formula worksheet helps compounders avoid variations in the compounding process by requiring the documentation of each ingredient, the quantity used, and providing the step-by-step process of assembling the compounded preparation. By conveying explicit instructions regarding the amount of time to mix a product, the quantity of the ingredients to add in and when, and the expected appearance, deviations from the norm can be avoided. SOPs should also be developed and enforced. SOPs describe the step-by-step process to complete a task and ensure that compounded medications are properly compounded, and equipment is appropriately maintained. There should be SOPs written for the following procedures at a minimum:

- Monitoring temperature
- Monitoring humidity
- Using any piece of equipment (electronic balance, pH meter or pH strips, hot plate, capsule machine) and assessment of calibration, if applicable
- Training personnel

- QC of test utilized throughout the compounding procedure (pH, bubble test, etc.)
- Testing of finished products via outside laboratories
- Labeling of compounded preparations

SOPs should be reviewed on a regular basis and updated as needed to reflect current processes and procedures. Is also important to ensure that everyone involved with compounding is aware what SOPs are available and when changes are made to those SOPs. Therefore, it is advisable to have a plan in place for where SOPs are located and how new SOPs and changes to existing SOPs will be communicated. This ensures that everyone knows what to expect and where to find the information.

In a veterinary clinic that is compounding medications, it is beneficial to complete some level of testing on finished preparations. This testing confirms that the procedure that is being followed and the techniques that are being used are accurate. Samples should periodically be sent to an outside laboratory to be assayed for potency. The documentation of this process and the results that are received serve as an additional QA/QC check. More information on types of testing available can be found in Chapter 3. For nonsterile products, any medications that have an extended BUD must be tested for antimicrobial effectiveness in its dispensing container at least once if there are not testing results available from an FDA-registered facility [1]. All other nonsterile compounds can be "spot-checked" as deemed necessary by the clinic and documented in their SOP. One option is to do a yearly spot check of a nonsterile preparation of each dosage form prepared by each person that is trained to compound. This will allow the identification of a potentially problematic process or a gap in training.

Mistakes will happen in any process where humans are involved, but the compounder should seek ways to prevent an error from occurring again instead of approaching the accident as a one-time occurrence. Errors should be looked at as a problem with a process and not a problem with the person. Initial QA and QC steps that can be implemented in the compounding process include checklists, checkpoints, requiring a second staff member to review calculations, integrating an automated software system, and individual ingredient descriptions among many other provisions. Additional methods for guaranteeing quality may be practice site specific and should be considered prior to offering compounding services as well as each time an error happens.

Labeling

Once the formulation is complete, it must be labeled appropriately following all state and federal regulations. Ensure that you adhere to all state-specific labeling requirements. However, in general, stock compounded preparations (e.g. those defined as anticipatory compounds) must contain the following labeling information [1, 2]:

- Assigned internal identification number, or lot number
- The active ingredient(s) and their quantity(ies), activity(ies), or concentration(s)
- Storage conditions (RT, refrigerated, frozen)
- BUD
- Dosage form
- Total amount of volume being prepared, if not visible or obvious in the container

Compounded preparations that are being dispensed to clients/patients should also include the following labeling information [1, 2]:

- Route of administration
- Indication for the compounded preparation

- Applicable special handling instructions
- Applicable warning statements
- The compounding facility name and contact information if being sent outside of the facility or healthcare system in which it was compounded (i.e. the name of and number for the practice/clinic)

As mentioned above, an SOP should be developed for the labeling of compounded products in order to prevent errors that may occur as well as prevent mix-ups of products. Products that are compounded also need to be differentiated from manufactured products by denoting within the drug name that it is compounded as discussed above. There may be specific wording designated by state regulations, and the compounder should verify that they are following applicable rules and regulations.

Packaging and Storage

Compounded medications must be packaged and stored appropriately following the USP. Packaging for each compounded preparation must be documented on the MFR. Selecting an appropriate container is dependent on the dosage form being compounded, the intended use of the compound, and the physical and chemical stability of the API(s) and excipient(s). As mentioned in Chapter 5, both the active ingredient(s) and excipient(s) have the risk of interacting with the container. Packaging materials may be reactive, or ingredients may adsorb to the material which can alter the characteristics of the compound including purity, strength, and quality. Therefore, if using extended stability data, the container must be the same as that used in the stability reference.

In the event that a USP monograph is not available, and no other sources have a formulation for a compounded product, pay special attention to the container that the manufactured product or bulk chemical is distributed in. Manufactured drugs that are packaged in an amber container typically require protection from light. Manufactured drugs that are packaged with excessive amounts of cotton are usually reactive to moisture. Manufactured drugs that are packed in glass containers are likely to interact with or contain an excipient that interacts with plastic. Many studies have also been completed on diluting manufactured products for humans, and those published studies (available from the American Society of Health-System Pharmacists (ASHP) Injectable Drugs Handbook and NCBI PubMed) can provide the compounder additional information on appropriate, as well as inappropriate, packaging, and storage. The ASHP Injectable Drugs Handbook is a resource for finding dilution and container computability information and will likely be easier to review since it is organized by drug.

Similar to manufactured medications, any chemicals that are utilized in the compounding process must be stored appropriately, as per the specifications in the monograph. This usually entails storage in a cool, dry place with the container closed tightly and protected from light; however, some chemicals may require refrigeration such as pluronic lecithin organogel. When determining where is appropriate to store manufactured medications or chemicals, it is important to keep in mind the following:

- Medications/drugs cannot be stored on the floor. Medications should be stored on shelving or in cabinets because storage on the floor can lead to contamination of medications, an example of adulteration, or lead to medications being broken.
- Manufactured medications should be removed from their boxes prior to storing in the compounding area/room. Boxes should not be brought into the compounding room as cardboard has been shown to contain mold spores. Removal of cardboard helps prevent potential contamination.

- Products that may be flammable or hazardous should be stored appropriately, away from other nonhazardous products. Drugs that are hazardous or flammable pose a significant risk of exposure to personnel handling them. To decrease the risk during handling and prevent cross-contamination, hazardous drugs should be stored in a designated area that is away from nonhazardous drugs. If a container were to break, it is preferred that this be away from other medications that may be contaminated.
- The storage area/room must meet temperature and humidity requirements provided in USP 795. As discussed in Chapter 5, the temperature and humidity in the area where compounding practices occur can have a significant effect on compounded preparations. Checking temperature and humidity daily and confirming that they are both within range helps ensure the quality of the preparations being compounded.

It is also advisable to have a temperature and humidity monitoring system in the storage area to identify any excursions that occur when no one is present. If a humidity spike occurs over a weekend, even if back to normal by Monday, that may have compromised the stability of active and inactive ingredients.

Additional information for packaging and storage requirements is available in USP 659.

Compounding Techniques

Trituration

Trituration is the process of reducing a powder's particle size. It is achieved through continuously grinding the powder in a mortar using a pestle. Difficulty of trituration depends on whether the drug that is being used for a compound is a manufactured product or an API. APIs are already in powder form and can be quickly triturated to ensure that the compounded product will be smooth and large pieces of powder will not form. Manufactured capsules can be opened, and the powder poured into a mortar. Usually, the powder is smooth and easy to triturate, but sometimes there may be larger bits present. It is good practice to triturate the powder for a quality compound regardless of the source.

Using manufactured tablets complicates the process a little. Tablets with a coating can be handled a couple ways. The coating does not incorporate into suspensions well, which leads some compounders to "wet" the tablet. This process involves wetting a paper towel and allowing the tablet to absorb a small amount of the moisture so that the outer coating can be rubbed off. This method may lead to slight loss of drug. Another process involves using a tablet splitter to break the tablet into smaller sections prior to trituration. This method can be followed up by using a sieve to sift out the larger pieces of coating that will be easily visible in the suspension. A third method involves soaking the tablets in a small amount of water (just enough to coat the tablets) for 5–10 minutes prior to trituration. This softens the tablet coating making it easier to crush. However, this method still incorporates the coating into the compound, which can result in stability issues. For coated tablets, it is important to use one of these methods as trying to crush the tablets in their original form may lead to breaking the mortar. Tablets without a coating should break down relatively easily by using the pestle to place slight pressure on them. In the case that a tablet is difficult to break down into powder form, a tablet splitter can be used to ease the process. It is important to note that all of these techniques may result in drug loss that could affect the final concentration. This potential loss should be considered when determining the best method.

Sifting

The process of sifting is very similar to sifting during the process of baking. Powder that contains larger pieces after trituration can be transferred to a weight boat. An appropriately sized sieve should then be place over top of the mortar as in Figure 6.3. Pouring small amounts of powder into the sieve and tapping it will allow the powder with an appropriate particle size through easily. This process will be continued until all of the powder from the weigh boat has been sifted. The larger pieces that remain can then be triturated in a separate mortar to reduce particle size appropriately.

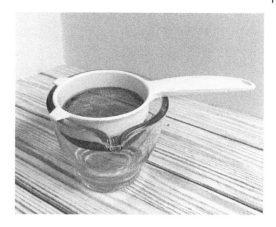

Figure 6.3 Sieve on mortar.

Sieves are made of thin metal; thus, if a spatula is used to spread the powder around, it should be plastic. If a metal spatula or other device is used, then small metal shavings can end up in the final product. Per USP, particles that are 75 μm or larger should be mechanically sieved. For smaller particles, sieving is not necessary, due to an insufficient amount of force. The process can actually cause particles to adhere to each other and to the sieve. The width of human hair to the width of paper is approximately equal to 75 μm.

Geometric Dilution

When mixing two ingredients that are not the same quantity, a special technique, geometric dilution, must be used to allow for thorough blending. Geometric dilution is utilized to dilute powders based on their measured quantities. Follow the below steps for appropriate incorporation of powders:

1) Ingredient 1 (smaller quantity) should be placed into the mortar
    a) Triturate alone if ingredient is nonmicronized or contains large clumps
    b) Sift ingredient if trituration does not provide appropriate particle size
2) Ingredient 2 (larger quantity) should be mixed into Ingredient 1 in small portions
    a) Add a portion of Ingredient 2 to 1 (in the mortar) that has the same volume of Ingredient 1, then thoroughly mix
    b) Then add a portion of Ingredient 2 to the combination in the mortar that has the same volume as the mixture, then thoroughly mix
    c) Complete mixing based upon the concept above in *Steps a + b* until Ingredient 2 is completely mixed into Ingredient 1
3) **Never** add the entire quantity of Ingredient 2 to 1 unless they are the same volume
    a) It is less likely that a uniform mixture will be achieved
    b) It will take a longer time period of mixing to achieve incorporation

Wetting

The process of wetting the powder prior to incorporation of the entire liquid vehicle is used to prevent large clumps from developing. Another term for a wetting agent is a levigating agent. The amount of wetting agent that is added into the compound depends upon the amount of powder in

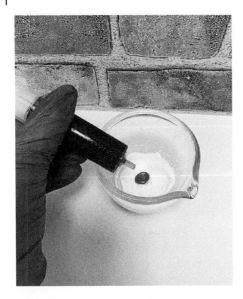

Figure 6.4 Small amount of vehicle to wet powder.

the mortar. Usually, a quantity around the size of a penny is sufficient (see Figure 6.4). Examples of wetting agents are glycerin, cthoxy diglycol, and propylene glycol. The liquid vehicle itself can also be used as a wetting agent though it does not improve solubility as other agents can. When incorporating the API and a liquid vehicle, developing a paste using a small amount of wetting agent not only avoids clumping of powders but can also improve the uniformity of the compounded preparation.

When the wetting agent is mixed with the powder in the mortar, the agent surrounds the powder and removes any surface air that is present to allow for the incorporation of insoluble and slightly soluble APIs. APIs that are soluble in the vehicle will not lose surface air until the dissolution process. An additional benefit to the wetting process is that friction leads to reduced particle size of the API.

Colored Tracers

The mixing of powders to be used for preparing a compounded capsule formulation can be improved by using a colored tracer. To avoid the potential for toxicity, natural powders, such as cyanocobalamin, should be used if possible. The tracer should be added to the API prior to adding other powdered ingredients. After the addition of the colored tracer, the process of geometric dilution must be followed for the remaining ingredients. Each time powder is added into the mortar, the components should be mixed until the tracer is evenly distributed throughout. Once all of the powdered ingredients are added and appropriately mixed, the colored tracer being appropriately dispersed confirms that the compounder can proceed to the next step in compounding capsules.

Equipment

Compounding medications requires a variety of equipment that is not normally kept in a veterinary clinic. There are also USP requirements that designate composition requirements for equipment as well as appropriate cleaning and sanitation practices. Appropriate equipment can be purchased from a variety of compounding wholesalers. Equipment must be of a composition that components that come into contact with the equipment surface will not be affected, and the material is not reactive, additive, or sorpitve [3]. This requirement ensures that the quality of your compounds, including purity, quality, and strength, will not be affected during the compounding process. Mortars and pestles are used for a variety of other tasks besides drug compounding such as preparing guacamole or grinding spices. They are so popular that you can purchase them on Amazon as well as from a variety of stores. The stone or granite mortar and pestle that may be utilized in culinary practices is not an acceptable material for compounding. Instead, glass or porcelain must be used.

Equipment should be stored in an appropriate place that protects it from being contaminated such as closed cabinets. Prior to completing any compounding, equipment that is to be used must be inspected for cleanliness, and the compounder must ensure that it is functioning correctly. Any equipment that is used to prepare hazardous products should preferably be dedicated for that use and stored separately from the other compounding equipment. If the clinic does not have the ability to store hazardous equipment separately, then disposable products can be used instead. If any nondisposable equipment is used for both hazardous and nonhazardous drugs (e.g. a counting tray), then there needs to be an SOP for how to clean the equipment after using for a hazardous drug.

Equipment must be washed with potable water, as described in the Environmental Protection Agency's National Primary Drinking Water Regulations (40 CFR Part 141) [4]. Compounding equipment can be hand-washed with soap and water or washed in a dishwasher with an appropriate detergent. If the clinic opts to utilize a dishwasher, it can only be used for compounding equipment, and care should be taken to ensure that all equipment washed this way is dishwasher safe. If the clinic opts to wash the dishes by hand, then they must utilize a drying rack or a lint-free towel to ensure that the items are completely dry. It is not recommended to use a blow dryer on compounding equipment in order to expedite the drying process as they have been shown to have a high level of bacterial contamination. The filter on a hair dryer only catches hair and other large particles like dust, which means any bacteria that have collected will be dispersed onto the compounding equipment. Though it is commonly found in most clinics, the use of isopropyl alcohol 70% as a cleaning agent for compounding equipment is not sufficient. Per USP definitions, isopropyl alcohol is a disinfectant and does not meet the standards for a cleaning agent. The standards require a cleaning agent to remove dirt, debris, microbes, and drug residues, and studies have shown that all of these criteria are not met, most evidently in the process of compounding hazardous products.

At a minimum, the following equipment is required for compounding otic medications:

– Oral syringes for administration by client (or dropper bottles for packaging)
– Containers of various sizes (amber oral liquid bottles)
– Appropriate auxiliary labels
– Injectable/oral syringes and needles for drawing up active ingredients from vials
– *Electronic balance*
– *Weigh boats/papers*
– *Spatulas/scoopulas/measuring spoons*

* Italicized items only needed if formula includes a medication in powder form

At a minimum, the following equipment is required for compounding solutions/suspensions:

– Mortar and pestles (glass versus ceramic)
– Graduated cylinders of various sizes
– Oral syringes for administration by client
– Containers of various sizes (amber oral liquid bottles)
– Appropriate auxiliary labels
– Injectable/oral syringes and needles for withdrawing ingredients from vials/bottles
– *Electronic balance*
– *Weigh boats/papers*
– *Spatulas/scoopulas/measuring spoons*

- *Syringe connectors (luer to luer, oral to oral, luer to oral)*
- *Sieve*
- *Beakers of various sizes*
- *pH paper*
- *Hot plate/stirring rod/stir bar*
- *Purified water dispenser*

* Italicized items only needed for particular formulas

At a minimum, the following equipment is required for compounding capsules:

- Mortar and pestles (glass versus ceramic)
- Electronic balance
- Weigh boats/papers
- Spatulas/scoopulas/measuring spoons
- Containers (pill bottles) of various sizes (drams)
- Appropriate auxiliary labels
- Empty gel capsules in appropriate size(s)
- *Capsule machine(s)*
- *Powder scraper/capsule stamper*

* Italicized items only needed for particular formulas

Selecting the appropriate equipment may seem daunting, but the following information should help.

Mortars and Pestles

A mortar and pestle can be purchased in varying sizes and varying materials. Glass mortars (see Figure 6.5) are considered to be advantageous to utilize when compounding as drugs do not typically adhere or absorb to them. They also cost less than ceramic mortars, are stain resistant, and work well with liquid compounds. Ceramic mortars are considered less fragile than glass mortars and notoriously are better for grinding chemicals down finely. For the preparation of emulsions, a more durable ceramic mortar and pestle with efficient "shearing" should be used. Overall, most compounders will choose glass mortars and utilize a sieve if they are concerned with particle size.

Maintaining stock with more than one mortar and pestle and in varying sizes is beneficial as it is not required to wash each piece of equipment prior to starting a new compound. Glass mortars are available in sizes that range from 2 to 32 oz. Recall from Chapter 5 that 1 oz is approximately equivalent to 30 ml, so a 2-oz mortar fits 60 ml and a 32-oz mortar fits 960 ml. However, this indicates that in a 2-oz

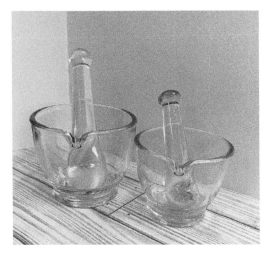

Figure 6.5 Mortars and pestles size 4 oz. (left) and 2 oz. (right).

mortar, 60 ml fits up to the top of the side. When compounding, it is appropriate to utilize the next largest size mortar if your quantity is greater than 75% of the mortar size.

Glassware

Glassware sizes (beakers and graduated cylinders) should also be taken into consideration depending on the preparations and quantities the clinic intends to prepare. A graduated cylinder is used to measure the volume of a liquid and has a narrow cylindrical shape (see Figure 6.6). Sizes range from 10 to 1000 ml. Reading a graduated cylinder has to be done at eye level in order to be accurate. This should be done by bending down to view it sitting on a flat surface versus holding it up to eye level, which is subject to inaccurate readings due to unintentional tilting. The center of the curve visible on the upper surface of the liquid, also known as the meniscus, is the measurement line. A beaker can also be used to measure the volume of liquid but is a container with a cylindrical shape and flat bottom like a cup (see Figure 6.7). Sizes range from 1 ml to several liters. When purchasing a beaker, it should be confirmed that it is graduated, meaning that it is marked on the side to indicate the volume contained. The marks, however, are not intended for precise measuring but instead are an estimate of the quantity. Both graduated cylinders and beakers typically have a small spout on the top for ease of pouring. When using glassware, the smallest size that is appropriate for measuring the quantity needed should be used. One way to confirm the accuracy of measurements with larger quantities is using two pieces of glassware (e.g. for measuring 206 ml, use a 200 mL and 10 ml graduated cylinder.) Graduated cylinders are far more accurate than beakers with a tolerance of ±1%, whereas beakers have an accuracy of up to ±10%. The use of a beaker for compounding requires appropriate calibration. A quantity of water can be measured using a graduated cylinder and then poured into the beaker. The meniscus should be marked on the beaker for appropriate measurements to confirm accuracy with use.

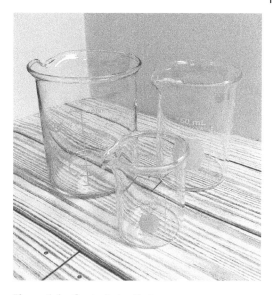

Figure 6.6 Graduated cylinders.

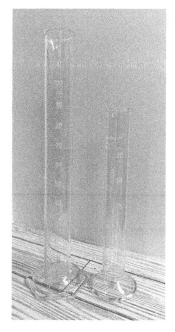

Figure 6.7 Beakers.

Containers

The container closure system that will be utilized must be documented on the MFR for each formulation. Drugs that are acidic tend to have little sorption to plastic, if any, but drugs that are basic can have substantial loss occur in plastic containers [3]. Examples of these drugs include

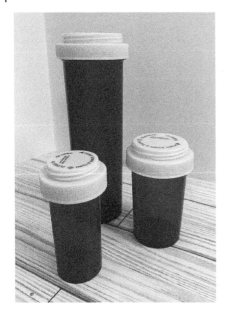

Figure 6.8 Varying sizes of drams.

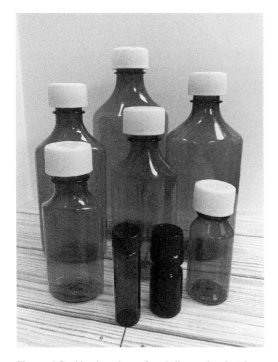

Figure 6.9 Varying sizes of oral dispensing bottles.

metoprolol, propranolol, and midazolam. Drugs that interact with plastic should be dispensed in glass containers and not be pulled up into syringes ahead of time. The only exception to this is if there is a stability study proving that drug concentration does not fall below 90% within a certain period of time for that compounded medication.

Plastic containers that provide ultraviolet (UV) protection for drugs denoting the need to protect from light include polyethylene terephthalate, polyvinyl chloride, and high-density polyethylene. Containers made of low-density polyethylene, polycarbonate, and polypropylene are not resistant to either part of the UV spectrum range or the entire UV spectrum [5]. Plastic and glass containers that protect medications from light are typically colored. Glass containers will be amber, whereas plastic containers can vary in color for tablet and capsules (see Figure 6.8) but will typically be amber/orange for liquid dispensing containers (see Figure 6.9).

Medications that are dispensed should be in a childproof container unless requested by the client otherwise. If the clinic does not have nonchildproof caps, they can examine their drams to determine if they have reversible caps (see above in Figure 6.8) or consider purchasing drams with reversible caps once their current stock runs out. Dispensing particular medications may require the use of a large bag, which is not tamper evident, but an appropriate auxiliary label denoting that the package is not child resistant meets requirements. Some containers available for use for compounded products may have a locking or tamper-evident cap. With tamper-evident containers, it is usually not possible to fit a stopper, a rubber insert (see Figure 6.10) that allows for the insertion of a syringe without leaking, which can make administration more difficult for the client. Good practice for any liquid medications includes dispensing with a stopper inserted into the bottle. Not only does it make administration easier for the client, but it can prevent potential spillage of medication and the need for the client to pick up a new prescription. If a stopper does not fit in the oral liquid container that is purchased, then the compounder can look into the option of "adaptacaps." Adaptacaps are a plastic cap with closure that can thread onto the bottle in place of the cap/top (see Figure 6.11).

The selection of an appropriately sized container for dispensing oral medications should be considered. Oral suspensions require being shaken prior to administration and, therefore, need enough space to allow for the resuspension of the compound. For both oral solutions and suspensions, it is important to not select too large of a container as there is potential for drug loss on the sides of the bottle. The larger the bottle dispensed, the more drug loss will occur. Capsules and tablets should not be overfilled in drams either. The overfilling of solid oral dosage forms can cause the client to spill the capsules or tablets upon opening the container or have problems reclosing the container without crushing the tablets/capsules.

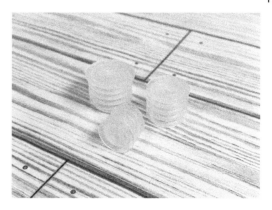

Figure 6.10 Oral dispensing inserts.

Scales

An electronic balance (see Figure 6.12) is utilized for weighing out powders, precisely. A Class A balance should be utilized for prescription compounding, and this differs from other classes based on sensitivity. However, 120 mg or less should not be weighed as it may have an error or 5% or more. In the case that a smaller weight is needed, a larger ingredient

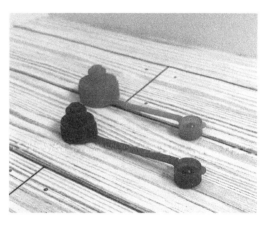

Figure 6.11 Adaptacaps.

of known weight should be mixed with the smaller ingredient and aliquoted for use [6]. This process involves the API and an inert powder like lactose. A ratio and proportion can be used to determine the weight of the API and inert powder that will be triturated together and the aliquot of the final mixture that needs to be used to make the compounded preparation. The weight of the API, inert drug, and weight of the aliquot all have to be >120 mg when using this method. The following equation should be used:

$$\frac{\text{Weight of API in mixture}}{\text{Weight of mixture}} = \frac{\text{Weight of API in aliquot}}{\text{Weight of aliquot}}.$$

If 6 mg of API is needed to prepare the compound, then the compounder will select a multiple of six that can be weighed with an appropriate degree of accuracy. The quantity must be increased to the minimum weight, 120 mg. The weight of aliquot can then be selected that will contain 6 mg of API

$$\frac{120\,\text{mg API}}{\text{Weight of mixture}} = \frac{6\,\text{mg API in aliquot}}{120\,\text{mg aliquot}}.$$

The completion of the calculation provides the total weight of the mixture, which is 2400 mg. This weight includes both the API and the inert drug. The weight of the inert drug,

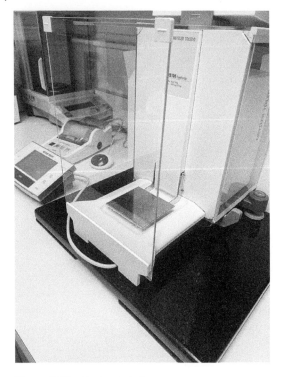

Figure 6.12 Electronic balance.

or diluent, can now be determined by subtracting the weight of the API from the total weight of the mixture.

$$2400 \text{ mg total} - 120 \text{ mg API}$$
$$= 2280 \text{ mg inert ingredient}$$

2280 mg of inert ingredient (i.e. lactose) would be added via geometric dilution to the 120 mg of API in order to allow for a 120-mg aliquot that contains 6 mg of API.

The largest quantity that can be weighed by a Class A balance is 120 g, but if this is not stated, then it should be assumed to be 15.5 g [6]. If the balance is not self-leveling/internal calibrating, then it should be tested to confirm that it meets the appropriate requirements as discussed in USP 1176. The compounder can complete routine checks to validate that their scale is performing appropriately using the provided manual; however, regular calibration should be completed by a service technician. The manual of the purchased scale will inform the user how often calibration is required. Once a place in the compounding area is selected for the scale, it should not be moved. A scale is calibrated for the precise location it is in at that time, and moving it will throw the calibration off. Units that have an internal calibration option can perform their own calibration automatically or whenever the compounder pushes the button to calibrate it. It can still be calibrated externally, and the authors recommend this as it may not calibrate the unit at full capacity, but it is not required. Calibration certificates should be maintained for all equipment that is calibrated as documented in the clinic's SOP.

A torsion balance (see Figure 6.13) was used for weighing powders prior to the electric balance and may still be used in practice by some compounders today. A torsion balance can be more durable and accurate than an electronic balance, but they require several steps in order to be appropriately calibrated. These steps can be time consuming and also lead to errors if they are done incorrectly. The smallest amount that is readable on a torsion balance is 120 mg. Knowing that the percent error in USP is ±5% for most formulas, you can find and/or confirm the least weighable quantity (LWQ). The LWQ is sensitivity divided by the percent error allowed all multiplied by 100%. The sensitivity, as discussed in Chapter 5, is the smallest amount of weight that can be added or removed before the dial moves one division. This is typically 6 mg, but there may be small variation

LWQ = 100% × (Sensitivity requirement/Acceptable error%)

LWQ = 100% × (6 mg/5%)

LWQ = 100% × 1.2 mg/%

LWQ = 120 mg.

Figure 6.13 Torsion balance. *Source:* Ref. [15].

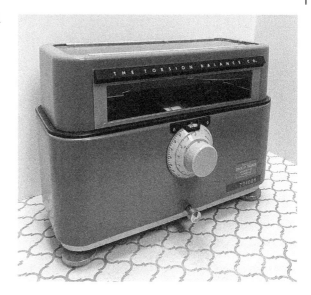

The torsion balance includes a set of weights for equilibration and calibration that are used in order to validate the sensitivity and weigh out correct quantities of powders. Both the torsion balance and the electronic balance are considered accurate, but there can be differences in sensitivity and readability. The readability is the smallest division at which the scale can be read (e.g. the number of places after the decimal point, 0.1–0.0000001 g). It tells the compounder the smallest amount that can be read on the scale, whereas sensitivity is the smallest amount of weight that causes a change in equilibrium or will cause the measurement to be detected. An electronic balance is likely to have better readability, but a torsion balance may have better sensitivity.

Spatulas and Measuring Devices

Spatulas and other measuring devices, for example, spoons and scoopulas, are available in plastic and stainless steel (see Figure 6.14). They can also be purchased as disposable plastic products. Both materials are used in different types of compounding practices. Plastic spatulas are used with chemicals that may interact with stainless steel blades. Drugs that are strong acids and bases are most likely to interact with stainless steel, while those that are weak acids and bases have no effect. Elements are added to steel in order to expand upon its properties, such as chromium and manganese. Metal chelators in large concentration should only be handled with plastic. Smaller stainless steel and plastic measuring devices are preferred for handling small amounts of powder, especially during the weighing. The compounder may find that they prefer to use plastic devices with liquids and creams and stainless steel with powders.

Equipment Cleaning

When or if additional equipment is purchased, such as a capsule machine or ointment mill, the manuals should be kept somewhere that is easily accessible, and an SOP should be developed for how they are used, if they require calibration, and how they should be cleaned. Larger equipment is cleaned using canned air or a lint-free cloth. Capsule machines should be appropriately washed between batches of capsules to remove any residue. The only exception to this is that if you are compounding capsules with the same drug but different strengths, you can start with the lower

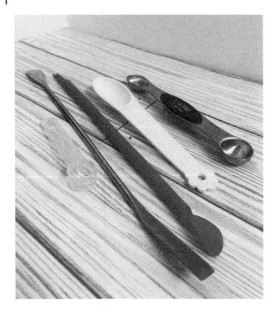

Figure 6.14 Varying types of spatulas.

strength of drug and then compound the higher strength of drug. The equipment used and the area where compounding occurs must be cleaned daily. The area where compounding is done must also be sprayed down with alcohol before and after any compounding occurs.

Specialty equipment that may be utilized in the compounding area includes an electric mortar and pestle (EMP) or an ointment mill. An EMP is a machine that efficiently and uniformly grinds down powders while mixing them. This machine can be very beneficial when making large batches of capsules. To ensure that appropriate mixing occurs, a colored powder tracer can be added to the mixture in the EMP or used in a standard mortar and pestle. An ointment mill utilizes high shearing force, which helps to disperse active ingredients homogenously throughout the product. There are three rollers that rotate in opposite directions and at different speeds in order to pull product through the gaps and decrease particle size. Ointment mills can also be utilized for creams and gels.

Training

Any personnel involved in the compounding process should be trained in the appropriate USP chapters. As previously mentioned, USP 795 covers nonsterile compounding, while USP 797 covers sterile compounding. In the event the practice compounds hazardous products, applicable USP 800 rules and regulations must also be incorporated into training. Topics that personnel should be trained on include QA, record keeping, equipment and supplies, hand hygiene, cleaning and sanitizing, measuring and mixing, understanding and interpreting safety data sheets (SDS), and reading and understanding procedures related to compounding and clinic specific formulation categories (e.g. otic medications, solutions, suspensions, capsules, etc.). After training is complete, personnel should feel comfortable with adhering to established standards of practice and documenting procedures appropriately. Figure 6.15 shows an example checklist for training.

Compounding is very similar to baking in that the wrong measurement or incorrect technique completely ruins the end product. For those new to compounding practice, it may be advantageous to compound preparations for an additional 10% in order to account for loss and guarantee that the client receives the total amount of medication that was prescribed. For example, when compounding trazodone 10 mg/ml suspension for a prescribed total of 100 ml, the formula would be prepared for 110 ml. The compounding process involves combining crushed tablets and a syrup-based vehicle in a mortar. Since the medication is compounded in a separate container, there may be slight loss on

USP 795 Nonsterile Compounding Training Checklist			
Training Topic	Expectations	Appropriately Trained (Y/N)	Additional Training Required
Hand Hygiene	• Location • Time • Procedure	☐ Yes ☐ No	1. 2.
Cleaning and Sanitizing	• Procedures • Cleaning Agents	☐ Yes ☐ No	1. 2.
Equipment and Supplies	• Calibration Procedures • Supplies to Use for Different Formulations	☐ Yes ☐ No	1. 2.
Measuring and Mixing	• Reading Liquid Volumes Using Meniscus • Mixing Procedures for all Components • Selecting Appropriate Mixing Vehicles	☐ Yes ☐ No	1. 2.
Record Keeping	• Documentation Requirements • SOPs	☐ Yes ☐ No	1. 2.
Quality Assurance	• SOP for QA Program • QC Initiatives	☐ Yes ☐ No	1. 2.
Understanding and Interpreting SDS	• SDS Location • Data Provided	☐ Yes ☐ No	1. 2.
Understanding Procedures for Clinic Specific Formulations	• Compounding Steps • Excipients • Species Specific Requirements	☐ Yes ☐ No	1. 2.

Figure 6.15   Compounding training checklist.

transfer during pouring or the sticky vehicle may stick to the glass mortar. When utilizing this method, it is important that all ingredients are increased by 10% and not just the vehicle.

The practice must also decide what their appropriate allowance is for their formulations. Most facilities use an allowance of ±5% of the expected concentration; yet, USP allows for ±10%. Facilities also have the option to have an even stricter allowance of ±3%. This must be documented in an SOP, followed by all personnel, and confirmed during a QA/QC check for each formula that is prepared. If the compounded medication that is prepared, such as a 10-mg capsules, is out of the expected range of the documented SOP but still within the ±10% allowance, then the SOP needs to be adjusted. This adjustment could be an allowance based on a particular number of capsules being out of the expected range but still within the USP allowance. It could also be that the compounder has to weigh double the number or all of the capsules to confirm that none of them are outside of the expected USP range.

Another important concept to cover during training is that each lot of drug and every product from a different manufacturer has the potential to behave differently. This is why it is crucial to complete packing statistics (see Chapter 5) when new product arrives as well as quantum satis (QS) on liquid formulations. If the usual product that is ordered is unavailable and a new manufacturer has to be used, the chemical may be denser, take up more space in the container, and require the use of fewer vehicles.

The humidity and temperature within the compounding area can also have an effect on chemicals. Per USP 659: Packaging and Storage Requirements, the humidity should not exceed 40% and the temperature should stay within the controlled room temperature range, 68–77 °F [7]. If an inorganic salt is being used for compounding, it can adsorb moisture in the air. This leads to differences in weight from what may be expected. When chemicals are not tightly sealed or are left open for extended periods of time, this can also have an effect. During capsule preparation, the active ingredient is often mixed with lactose to create the appropriate strength of medication. However, on days with high humidity or high temperature, the lactose may become "fluffier" or denser. In the event that the compounding area has a tendency to be too humid, a dehumidifier should be purchased.

Formulation Instructions

The MF and CR require step-by-step instructions for how the compound is prepared. The instructions have to be detailed enough to be easily repeatable yet not be convoluted. Instructions will differ depending on the formulation made, but the steps below provide a starting point that can be further adjusted to meet the clinic's specifications.

<u>Preparing an otic medication</u> (Example = Enrofloxacin/Synotic (1:2) Compounded Otic [see Figure 6.16])

1) Calculate the ingredient amounts that will be used and record the calculations
2) Draw up liquids into appropriately sized syringes/glassware, weight out any powders and record weight(s)
3) *Formulation specific*
   a) Liquid + powder: Place powder in a mortar and triturate into a fine powder (to step 4)
   b) Liquid only: Place ingredients into appropriately sized dispensing bottle (to step 7)

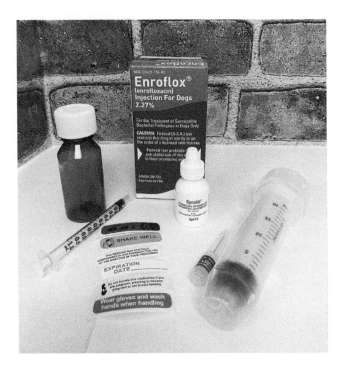

Figure 6.16 Equipment and ingredients for enrofloxacin/synotic (1:2) compounded otic.

4) Add a small amount of wetting agent to powder and mix into a smooth paste
5) Add enough of your vehicle to transform the paste into a liquid and transfer to a dispensing bottle
   a) Using a plastic spatula, scrape out as much of liquid residue as possible from mortar and transfer to dispensing bottle
6) Add any remaining vehicle to the dispensing bottle and shake well
7) Label with prescription label, the appropriate auxiliary labels, and dispense with oral syringe(s) or dropper

Preparing a solution (Example = Calcitriol 0.1-mg/ml Compounded Oral Solution [see Figure 6.17])

1) Calculate the ingredient amounts that will be used and record the calculations
2) Draw up liquids into appropriately sized syringes/glassware
3) Place ingredients into appropriately sized oral dispensing bottle and shake well
4) Label with prescription label, the appropriate auxiliary labels, and dispense with oral syringe(s)

Preparing a suspension (Example = Trazodone 10-mg/ml Compounded Oral Suspension [see Figure 6.18])

1) Calculate the ingredient amounts that will be used and record the calculations
2) Count out tablets needed, draw up liquids into appropriately sized syringes/glassware, and weight out any additional powders and record weight(s)
   a) *If using API: weigh out powder and record weight*
3) Place tablets/API in a mortar and triturate into a fine powder

Figure 6.17 Equipment and ingredients for calcitriol 0.1-mg/ml compound.

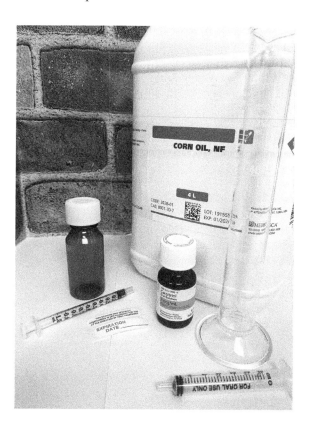

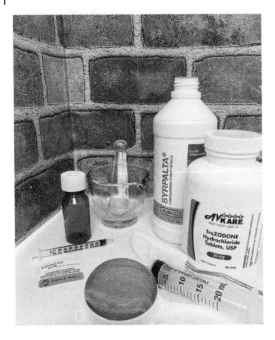

Figure 6.18 Equipment and ingredients for trazodone 10-mg/ml compounded suspension.

4) If bitterness reducing powder or flavor powder is requested, add to mortar and triturate with drug powder
5) Add a small amount of wetting agent to powder and mix into a smooth paste
6) Add enough of your vehicle to transform the paste into a liquid and transfer to an oral dispensing bottle
   a) Using a plastic spatula, scrape out as much of liquid residue as possible from mortar and transfer to oral dispensing bottle
7) Add any remaining vehicle to the oral dispensing bottle and shake well
   a) QS if denoted in the formula
8) Label with prescription label, the appropriate auxiliary labels, and dispense with oral syringe(s)

Preparing a transdermal medication (Example = Amlodipine 4.17-mg/ml Compounded Transdermal)

1) Calculate the ingredient amounts that will be used and record the calculations
2) Weigh out powder(s) and record weight(s)
3) Add powder(s) to mortar and triturate
4) Add a small amount of wetting agent to powder and mix into a smooth paste
5) Add ~50% of vehicle and with paste until appropriately combined
6) Transfer the mixture to an appropriate size syringe using a plastic spatula
   a) Using plastic spatula, scrape out as much of residue as possible from mortar and transfer to syringe
   b) To transfer, pull out plunger and backfill syringe
7) Add plunger back into syringe **carefully** until you hear it click
8) Tap the bottom of the plunger on the counter to allow built up pressure to release from the syringe
9) Once pressure is released, **carefully** push plunger until you can determine an accurate amount of product in syringe

10) Following steps 6–9 backfill a second syringe of the same size until quantity as denoted on the prescription is reached
    a) QS if denoted in the formula
11) Connect syringes using an appropriate connector (luer to luer, luer to slip, slip to slip) and mix well moving the compound between syringes until uniform
    a) Mix for 3 minutes to ensure uniformity
12) Push compound into one syringe and disconnect connector and second syringe
13) Tap plunger on the counter until there are no air pockets present
14) Transfer to smaller, oral syringes (1 ml)
    a) Remove plunger from 1 ml syringes and backfill by place tip of syringe containing product in the back of the 1 ml syringe
    b) Slowly push compound into 1 ml syringe until syringes is full
    c) When adding plunger back to syringe, insert at an angle to prevent air pockets
    d) Tap plunger of 1 ml syringe on counter to confirm there are no air pockets
    e) Push any extra drug not required for dose back into the syringe containing the large amount of product
15) Repeat step 14 until all syringes are full
16) Label each syringe with patient information and place in dispensing bag with prescription label and appropriate auxiliary labels

Preparing capsules

1) Calculate the ingredient amounts that will be used and record the calculations
2) Count out tablets needed, draw up liquids into appropriately sized syringes/glassware, and Weigh out powder(s) and record weight(s)
3) Add powder(s) to mortar and triturate, using geometric dilution
4) Load capsule machine with appropriately sized capsules
5) Using machine, remove tops of capsules and drop into place so they are flush with the top plate
6) Add mixed powder in small quantities
    a) Do not add powder in the middle of the machine every time
7) Once all powder has been evenly distributed, add tops of capsules back using machine
8) Remove capsules by unlocking machine and pulling off top section
9) Prior to dumping capsules out, they must be locked into place by lightly pressing down onto each individual capsule
10) Remove any excess powder from capsules using lint-free cloth
11) Weight out 10 capsules, record weights, and confirm they meet acceptable strength range designated by clinic
12) Count number of capsules requested by prescription, pour into appropriately sized dram, and label with prescription label and appropriate auxiliary labels

Species-Specific Information

Flavoring

There are particular flavoring types that some species tend toward; however, it can sometimes be trial and error. Every animal has their favorite foods or snacks, and compounded medication administration is made much easier if the medication tastes like something that they enjoy. Cats and dogs usually prefer meat flavors or flavors associated with pet treats like cheese and peanut butter. Oddly enough, both species also enjoy marshmallow flavor either alone or in combination with other flavors. The thought behind why marshmallow is popular in veterinary patients is due to it decreasing the bitterness of medication and making a more palatable flavor. Pocket pets tend to prefer sweeter flavors. Based on the authors' pocket pet patient population, you cannot go wrong with tutti frutti. Ferrets that do not like sweet flavors usually enjoy meat-based flavors like bacon and beef. Exotic patients also have a preference toward sweet flavors as do horses.

As discussed in previous chapters, flavoring is available in liquid and powder form. Liquid flavoring may be available in an aqueous formulation, such as Flavorx products that are water soluble, or nonaqueous like cod liver oil. Liquid, aqueous flavoring should be utilized in aqueous formulations, while nonaqueous liquid flavoring or powder flavors should be utilized in oil-based formulations. If preferred, powder flavors can be used for both aqueous and nonaqueous formulations.

The list in Table 6.1 is not all inclusive but can be used to select a handful of flavors to be used for compounding for a variety of species.

Toxicities

Examples of toxicities for excipients were discussed in Chapter 5. Table 6.2 provides additional products or chemicals that may be included in compounding formulations. Cats have a limited ability to glucuronidate, meaning that they cannot eliminate toxic metabolites from products that require conjugation with glucuronide. This deficiency is not generalized to all glucuronidated drugs though. It is dependent upon drug structure, and an increased toxicity is seen with the simple planar phenolic structure. Azo dyes, the artificial colors commonly used in food and drugs, contain phenolic moieties. If a colored tracer is used for capsules or powders when preparing formulations for cats, the compounder should confirm that it is not classified as an azo dye or look up the chemical structure to confirm no phenolic structures are present. Cats

Table 6.1 Species-specific flavoring options.

Species	Flavor
Small animal	
Cats	Bacon, beef, cheese, chicken, cod liver oil, fish, marshmallow, tuna
Dogs	Bacon, beef, cheese, chicken, peanut butter, liver, marshmallow
Pocket pets	
Ferrets	Apple, bacon, beef, peanut butter, orange, raspberry, strawberry, tutti frutti
Guinea pigs	Apple, fish, orange, raspberry, strawberry, tuna, tutti frutti
Rabbits	Banana, raspberry, strawberry, tutti frutti
Rats/mice	Banana, orange, raspberry, strawberry, tutti frutti
Exotics	
Birds	Apple, banana, grape, orange, raspberry, strawberry, tutti frutti
Reptiles	Banana, orange, tutti frutti
Large animal	
Horses	Apple, alfalfa, caramel, maple, molasses

Table 6.2 Species-specific toxicities in compounding formulations.

Product/chemical	Toxicity
Cats	
Alcohols	Depression of CNS, hypoglycemia [7]
Azo dyes (artificial colors)	Methemoglobinemia [8, 9]
Benzoic acid derivatives (benzyl alcohol)	Excessive CNS stimulation, hemolytic anemia, methemoglobinemia [7, 9]
Propylene glycol	Hemolytic anemia (Heinz body anemia) [9]
Dogs	
Alcohol	Depression of CNS [7]
Chocolate	Excessive cardiovascular and CNS stimulation [7]
Cremophor	Anaphylaxis from too much histamine release [10]
Polysorbate 80	Anaphylaxis from too much histamine release [11]
Xylitol	Hypoglycemia from too much insulin release [7]
Birds	
Chocolate	Anaphylaxis from too much histamine release [12]
Xylitol	Hypoglycemia from too much insulin release [13]

experience the same metabolic problem with benzoic acid derivatives along with amino acid conjugation with glycine. Alcohols and propylene glycol can result in serious toxicities in cats; however, this typically occurs from exposure to larger quantities. Propylene glycol is commonly used as a "wetting agent," where a small amount is introduced into powdered drug to help with the incorporation of powder into the liquid vehicle. Though this amount is not enough to cause toxicity, best practice would be to switch the wetting agent to glycerin or ethoxy diglycol since these are both acceptable wetting agents without the toxicity concern. While either glycerin or ethoxy diglycol can be used, the authors' preference is ethoxy diglycol due to a stickier consistency produced when using glycerin.

Alcohol in dogs can also lead to serious toxicities, typically following a short period of excitement. Chocolate contains two different methylxanthines, which result in increased cardiovascular and central nervous system (CNS) stimulation. The toxicity is dose related, and though artificial chocolate does not have the same toxicity, it should be avoided to prevent dogs from becoming interested in the true product. When given to dogs, Cremophor, polysorbate 20, and polysorbate 80 can all lead to an excess of histamine being released in a short period of time, causing anaphylaxis. All three of these ingredients are nonionic surfactants and cause a decrease in systemic vascular resistance and vasodilation, which is related to histamine release [14]. The toxicity is far worse when the products are given via injectable routes but can still lead to severe gastrointestinal upset and pruritis when given via other routes of administration. Xylitol is not typically found in compounding formulas due to the knowledge we have required regarding toxicities, but it may be present in manufactured products. Xylitol is a sugar alcohol that is absorbed much quicker in dogs and causes a rapid release of insulin from the pancreatic beta cells, leading to severe hypoglycemia and, at higher doses, potential hepatotoxicity. Therefore, avoiding xylitol in commercial formulations may be a reason to utilize a compounded medication.

Birds experience similar toxicities as dogs to chocolate and xylitol [12, 13], so these products should be avoided in their compounded products. In the compounding world, it has long been thought that birds could not be given oil-based oral products (solutions, suspensions). Reasons for this vary and include birds being coated with oil preening themselves and losing the ability to thermoregulate as well as organ damage, the risk of hypertriglyceridemia, and the risk of aspiration. However, the volume of compounded nonaqueous products that birds receive is negligible, which often decreases these concerns allowing for the compounder to provide a wider array of compounded products for our feathered friends. This is a case where risk versus benefit should be considered when determining if a compound should be prepared in an aqueous or oil vehicle.

Potency Designations

APIs, the bulk drugs used for compounding, are not always considered to be 100% potent. APIs can have their potency expressed in a variety of forms including activity, micrograms per milligram, and units of activity. When considering drug potency, there is a reference standard that has been used in comparison, which is why some drugs are expressed as a range. Overall, it refers to the relative strengths of APIs that can give the same effect. The potency of a drug is often measured on a dried or anhydrous basis as opposed to an "as is" basis. This can be drug specific though and is dependent on the standard included in the USP monograph for the drug. If the potency is measured on a dried or anhydrous basis, this will be noted on the CoA. If nothing is noted, then it was measured "as is." Regardless of how the potency is measured, it is paramount to keep the container tightly closed and in a dry storage area.

If the potency of the CoA is noted as anhydrous, then it does not include water. If the water content is high on the CoA, then it should be included in the calculations. The water content must be subtracted from the drug in order to determine the actual potency of the drug. The following equation shows the process of completing potency calculations based on the CoA assay for a drug being 99.6% (anhydrous drug) with a water content of 4.8%:

$$\frac{100\% - \text{Water content}\left(\text{CoA}\right)}{100} = \text{Quantity of water free drug}$$

$$\frac{\text{Quantity of water free drug} \times \text{Assay}\%}{100} = \text{Potency of drug}$$

$$\frac{100\% - 4.8\%}{100} = 0.952$$

$$\frac{0.952 \, x \, 99.6\%}{100} = 0.948.$$

After determining the potency, it can be used to determine the amount of drug needed for the compound. The amount of drug needed is divided by the potency, and the answer equals the amount of drug needed for the compound.

If the API is in a salt form, then the potency designation may include the salt; otherwise, it is normally established from the base of the drug (e.g. doxycycline monohydrate established on doxycycline only). The label on the API will have values on it that will be needed for any calculations prior to compounding the product. Potency may be mistakenly considered the same as strength, but they do not describe the same thing. Potency focuses on the effect of a drug and how that effect relates to different drugs that are able to produce a similar effect. The strength of a medication does not describe the drug's effect. The example below shows how to utilize the potency provided on an APIs label.

A compounding formula requires a total of 26 mg of amlodipine besylate. You receive the API, and the label states the following, "80 μg of amlodipine per mg of powder." As the potency is expressed as micrograms per milligram, you will need to complete a calculation to determine the quantity of powder to provide 25 mg of amlodipine besylate.

$$\frac{80\,\mu g}{1000\,\mu g} = \frac{26\,mg}{X}$$

$$X = 325\,mg$$

Upon the completion of the calculation, it can be determined that 325 mg of powder is needed to provide 26 mg of actual amlodipine besylate. This concept is similar to how if a compounder were to weigh at 2.5 mg tablet of amlodipine besylate, it would weigh more than 2.5 mg due to the addition of excipients.

Feasibility for a Veterinary Clinic

Introducing the practice of compounding into a veterinary clinic is not as big of an undertaking as it may seem. There is an upfront cost for equipment, access to formulas, and ingredients, but it has the potential to pay for itself many times over. Depending on the formulas, the clinic intends to prepare many of the vehicles, and excipients can be utilized for a multitude of compounds. Preparing compounded medications in house may also lead to better relationships with clients as nobody wants to hear their pet has a condition that requires treatment, but that treatment has to be shipped to them and cannot be started for three to five days.

There is also time that is required during the initial phase of compounding practice. However, a lot of the documentation like SOPs can be purchased from reputable companies, or examples can be found online to provide a general framework. Training programs are also available from a variety of sources. This would allow the "responsible person" to complete a training program and then train the remainder of the staff that would be involved in compounding practices.

Preparing compounded medication in house provides those who work in the clinic a sense of comfortability because they know the patients and they develop relationships with and take care of are receiving quality medication. For the responsible person to establish compounding in practice, they should follow the below steps.

1) Designate an area in the practice for nonsterile compounding
2) Develop a list of formulations the practice plans to prepare
3) Review all USP standards and state regulations that pertain to each planned compound
4) Consider a hands-on training course to further solidify the concepts covered in this book
5) Prepare appropriate documentation for each compound (MFR and CR)
6) Write SOPs for nonsterile compounding processes
7) Purchase appropriate ingredients and equipment for nonsterile compounding
8) Develop training checklist for nonsterile compounding
9) Prepare formulations on compounding list to confirm they work out as expected
10) Train staff appropriately using training checklist
11) Compound quality medications for your patients

References

1 USP (2023). *USP General Chapter <795> Pharmaceutical Compounding – Nonsterile Preparations.* Rockville, MD: USP.

2 USP (2019). *USP General Chapter <795> Pharmaceutical Compounding – Nonsterile Preparations.* Rockville, MD: USP.

3 Palmgrén, J.J., Mönkkönen, J., Korjamo, T. et al. (2006). Drug adsorption to plastic containers and retention of drugs in cultured cells under in vitro conditions. *Eur. J. Pharm. Biopharm.* 64 (3): 369–378. https://doi.org/10.1016/j.ejpb.2006.06.005. Epub 2006 Jun 29. PMID: 16905298.

4 USP (2017). *USP General Chapter <661> Plastic Packaging Systems and Their Materials of Construct.* Rockville, MD: USP.

5 USP (2022). *USP General Chapter <1176> Pharmaceutical Compounding – Prescription Balances and Volumetric Apparatus.* Rockville, MD: USP.

6 USP (2017). *USP General Chapter <659> Pharmaceutical Compounding – Packaging and Storage Requirements.* Rockville, MD: USP.

7 Kovalkovičová, N., Sutiaková, I., Pistl, J., and Sutiak, V. (2009). Some food toxic for pets. *Interdiscip. Toxicol.* 2 (3): 169–176. https://doi.org/10.2478/v10102-009-0012-4. Epub 2009 Sep 28. PMID: 21217849; PMCID: PMC2984110.

8 Kobylewski, S. and Jacobson, M.F. (2012). Toxicology of food dyes. *Int. J. Occup. Environ. Health* 18 (3): 220–246. https://doi.org/10.1179/1077352512Z.00000000034 PMID: 23026007.

9 Javinsky, E. (2012). Hematology and immune-related disorders. *The Cat* 643–703. https://doi.org/10.1016/B978-1-4377-0660-4.00025-9. Epub 2011 Dec 5. PMCID: PMC7271196.

10 Stokes, A.H., Kemp, D.C., Faiola, B. et al. (2013). Effects of Solutol (Kolliphor) and cremophor in polyethylene glycol 400 vehicle formulations in Sprague-Dawley rats and beagle dogs. *Int. J. Toxicol.* 32 (3): 189–197. https://doi.org/10.1177/1091581813485452. Epub 2013 Apr 24. PMID: 23616145.

11 Holbrook, K., Andrews, D., Sutherland, W. et al. (2022). Threshold for anaphylactoid reaction to polysorbate 80 in canines. *Int. J. Toxicol.* 41 (2): 89–98. https://doi.org/10.1177/10915818211063478. Epub 2022 Mar 25. PMID: 35337210.

12 Gartrell, B.D. and Reid, C. (2007). Death by chocolate: a fatal problem for an inquisitive wild parrot. *N. Z. Vet. J.* 55 (3): 149–151. https://doi.org/10.1080/00480169.2007.36759. PMID: 17534419.

13 Gardner, B.R. and Mitchell, E.P. (2017). Acute, fatal, presumptive xylitol toxicosis in cape sugarbirds (*Promerops cafer*). *J. Avian Med. Surg.* 31 (4): 356–358. https://doi.org/10.1647/2016-234. PMID: 29327962.

14 Johnson, R.A., Simmons, K.T., Fast, J.P. et al. (2011). Histamine release associated with intravenous delivery of a fluorocarbon-based sevoflurane emulsion in canines. *J. Pharm. Sci.* 100 (7): 2685–2692. https://doi.org/10.1002/jps.22488. Epub 2011 Jan 18. PMID: 21246564; PMCID: PMC3102263.

15 The Torsion Balance Co. https://www.chem-rg.com/listings/1488252-used-vintage-torsion-dlt2-balance-120g-x-0-01g (accessed 13 January 2023).

Index

Please note that page references to Figures will be followed by the letter 'f', to Tables by the letter 't'

Drug Compounding for Veterinary Professionals, First Edition. Lauren R. Eichstadt Forsythe and Alexandria E. Gochenauer.
© 2023 John Wiley & Sons, Inc. Published 2023 by John Wiley & Sons, Inc.
Companion Website: www.wiley.com/go/forsythe/drug